2005

Roger B. Fillingim, PhD

Concise Encyclopedia
of Pain Psychology

Pre-publication
REVIEWS,
COMMENTARIES,
EVALUATIONS . . .

"*Concise Encyclopedia of Pain Psychology* is literally pain psychology from A to Z. Dr. Fillingim has done a masterful job of capturing the essence of many of the psychological terms and concepts as they relate to pain. The references are well-selected and up-to-date. This book would be of great value to the novice and experienced researcher, clinician, and academician. For the psychologically trained and, perhaps even more so, for the nonpsychologically trained, this is a useful reference and guide. It could be especially helpful to those preparing for board-type examinations."

Daniel M. Doleys, PhD
Director, Pain and Rehabilitation
Institute, The Doleys Clinic,
Birmingham, Alabama

"The biopsychosocial model serves as the foundation of this book. Research has increasingly emphasized the need to integrate 'mind and body' when understanding pain. This is an excellent resource book for the novice in pain psychology as well as the seasoned clinician. Physicians will also appreciate this book as a reference tool, which provides a brief literature review on a variety of pain topics. Dr. Fillingim includes an extensive reference section specific to each topic presented in the book. He provides bottom-line conclusions, usually in less than two pages. These brief summaries can be efficient tools for the busy clinician, who has little time to read the original publications."

Virgil T. Wittmer, PhD
Director of Pain Rehabilitation,
Brooks Rehabilitation,
Jacksonville, Florida

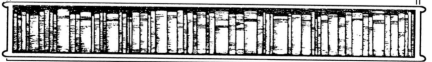

More pre-publication
REVIEWS, COMMENTARIES, EVALUATIONS . . .

"**P**ain is an unpleasant subjective experience produced by a complex interaction of physiologic, psychological, and social factors. Optimal assessment and treatment of persistent pain, then, requires the expertise of pain psychologists who interact effectively with physicians and other health professionals as well as with patients. Dr. Fillingim has produced a comprehensive and highly readable resource that surveys the major constructs and methods of assessment and treatment used by professionals in the field of pain psychology. The *Concise Encyclopedia of Pain Psychology* provides clear definitions and brief reviews of the scientific literature concerning these constructs and methods. This volume will be a highly valuable text for trainees and postgraduate professionals in the medical or health sciences who provide interdisciplinary care to patients with persistent pain. It will greatly enhance communication among these health professionals and foster improved patient care."

Laurence A. Bradley, PhD
Professor of Medicine, Division of Clinical Rheumatology and Immunology, University of Alabama at Birmingham

"**T**o my knowledge this is the first book that has attempted to provide an encyclopedia of terms in pain psychology. This book is long overdue and will be enormously useful to individuals who need a greater understanding of the broad field of pain psychology. It will be especially appealing to pain practitioners who are not psychologists, but who frequently interact with pain psychologists. It will also be quite helpful to a range of students who have interests in pain psychology.

This book is clearly written and well-organized. It is much more than a dictionary or taxonomy of terms in pain psychology. Each entry provides a brief review that includes recent key paper citations. These citations are up-to-date and provide an excellent starting point for anyone who wants to pursue a more in-depth review of a topic."

Francis J. Keefe, PhD
Professor, Psychiatry and Behavioral Sciences; Director, Pain Prevention and Treatment Program, Duke University Medical School

More pre-publication
REVIEWS, COMMENTARIES, EVALUATIONS . . .

"This book fills an important void in the published literature by providing a brief, yet comprehensive and informative, review of important topics and terms that serve as the basis of the field of pain psychology, and in fact, for the field of pain and pain management, more broadly. The volume is uniquely formatted and includes two primary components. Following a brief and thoughtful introduction to the volume, Dr. Fillingim provides an alphabetized consideration of the most common constructs employed in the field. The discussion of each topic incorporates a selective and scholarly consideration of important clinical and research issues. The discussions are easy to understand and capture the central issues related to each topic. A particular strength of this section is the fact that it incorporates references to both landmark publications in the field and to more recent publications that represent the state-of-the-art theory, science, and clinical thinking.

The book is clearly a testament to Dr. Fillingim's extraordinary scholarship and breadth and depth of knowledge of this large and continually expanding field of inquiry and clinical importance. Ultimately, *Concise Encyclopedia of Pain Psychology* is likely to serve a novel role in defining the field of pain psychology and as an important resource for pain specialists and for other clinicians and scholars alike."

Robert D. Kerns, PhD
Professor of Psychiatry, Neurology,
and Psychology, Yale University;
Chief, Psychology Service,
VA Connecticut Healthcare System;
National Consultant for Pain Management,
Department of Veterans Affairs

The Haworth Medical Press®
The Haworth Reference Press™
Imprints of The Haworth Press, Inc.
New York • London • Oxford

Concise Encyclopedia
of Pain Psychology

THE HAWORTH MEDICAL PRESS®
Titles of Related Interest

Psychotherapy and the Somatizing Patient edited by E. Mark Stern and Virginia Fraser Stern

Fibromyalgia, Chronic Fatigue Syndrome, and Repetitive Strain Injury: Current Concepts in Diagnosis, Management, Disability, and Health Economics edited by Andrew Chalmers, Geoffrey Owen Littlejohn, Irving E. Salit, and Frederick Wolfe

Lost Voices: Women, Chronic Pain, and Abuse by Nellie A. Radomsky

Disease, Pain, and Suicidal Behavior by Elsebeth Stenager and Egon Stenager

Autogenic Training: A Mind-Body Approach to the Treatment of Fibromyalgia and Chronic Pain Syndrome by Micah R. Sadigh

Minding the Body: Psychotherapy in Cases of Chronic and Life-Threatening Illness edited by Ellyn Kaschak

The Concise Encyclopedia of Fibromyalgia and Myofascial Pain by Roberto Patarca-Montero

The Psychopathology of Functional Somatic Syndromes: Neurobiology and Illness Behavior in Chronic Fatigue Syndrome, Fibromyalgic, Gulf War Illness, Irritable Bowel, and Premenstrual Dysphoria by Peter Manu

Concise Encyclopedia of Pain Psychology

Roger B. Fillingim, PhD

The Haworth Medical Press®
The Haworth Reference Press™
Imprints of The Haworth Press, Inc.
New York • London • Oxford

For more information on this book or to order, visit
http://www.haworthpress.com/store/product.asp?sku=5416

or call 1-800-HAWORTH (800-429-6784) in the United States
and Canada or (607) 722-5857 outside the United States and Canada

or contact orders@HaworthPress.com

Published by

The Haworth Medical Press® and The Haworth Reference Press™, imprints of The Haworth Press, Inc., 10 Alice Street, Binghamton, NY 13904-1580.

PUBLISHER'S NOTE
This book has been published solely for educational purposes and is not intended to substitute for the medical advice of a treating physician. **Medicine is an ever-changing science. As new research and clinical experience broaden our knowledge, changes in treatment may be required. While many potential treatment options are made herein, some or all of the options may not be applicable to a particular individual. Therefore, the author, editor, and publisher do not accept responsibility in the event of negative consequences incurred as a result of the information presented in this book. We do not claim that this information is necessarily accurate by the rigid scientific and regularity standards applied for medical treatment.** No warranty, expressed or implied, is furnished with respect to the material contained in this book. The reader is urged to consult with his/her personal physician with respect to the treatment of any medical condition.

Cover design by Jennifer M. Gaska.

Library of Congress Cataloging-in-Publication Data

Fillingim, Roger B., 1962-
    Concise encyclopedia of pain psychology / Roger B. Fillingim.
        p. cm.
    Includes index.
    ISBN-13: 978-0-7890-1893-9 (hc. : alk. paper)
    ISBN-10: 0-7890-1893-4 (hc. : alk. paper)
    ISBN-13: 978-0-7890-1894-6 (pbk. : alk. paper)
    ISBN-10: 0-7890-1894-2 (pbk. : alk. paper)
    1. Pain—Encyclopedias. 2. Pain—Psychological aspects—Encyclopedias. I. Title.

RB127.F55 2005
616'.0472'03—dc22

                                                                        2004027194

CONTENTS

ABOUT THE AUTHOR

Roger B. Fillingim, PhD, is an associate professor at the University of Florida, College of Dentistry, and a staff psychologist with the North Florida/South Georgia VA Health System. He has published numerous articles and book chapters, and edited the books *Sex, Gender, and Pain* and *Pathophysiology of Pain Perception* (with S. Lautenbacher). He currently serves on the editorial boards of the journals *Pain, XXvsXY (3XY): The International Journal of Sex Differences in the Study of Health and Disease in Aging, The Journal of Pain,* and *Psychosomatic Medicine.* He is the recipient of multiple grants from the National Institutes of Health and is a frequent speaker at national and international meetings. He is a member of the American Pain Society, the American Psychosomatic Society, the International Association for the Study of Pain, and the Society of Behavioral Medicine. For the past several years, Dr. Fillingim's research has focused on understanding the nature of individual differences in pain and analgesia, such as the complex biopsychosocial factors underlying sex-related and ethnic influences on pain, and he is an internationally recognized expert in this field.

Introduction

This book is a resource of terms, definitions, classic papers, and important findings related to the field of pain psychology. The first term that requires definition is pain psychology itself. Pain psychology refers to the application of psychological principles and methods to enhance the understanding of pain. This broad definition subsumes the clinical, conceptual, and scientific components of pain psychology. As a professional discipline, pain psychology is not an officially recognized subspecialty in psychology; however, it is informally acknowledged as an important area of expertise. The field of pain psychology has a long history, and its scientific and clinical contributions in the area of pain management have grown exponentially over the past several decades. Indeed, at this time, pain psychologists are an integral part of the multidisciplinary approach to pain evaluation and treatment. Moreover, pain psychology encompasses a wide range of both scientific and clinical endeavors.

In order to provide a context for this book, I suggest three guiding principles that form the foundation for pain psychology. First, mind-body dualism must be abandoned—really. Despite the tremendous advances in understanding the neurobiology of pain, including important findings documenting that psychological variables produce direct neurobiological influences on pain, artificial distinctions between biological and psychosocial contributions persist. Indeed, distinctions between "psychosocial" and "biological" factors are based more on the level of analysis than actual mechanisms of action. For example, at a psychosocial level, expectations may alter pain responses, while from a more biological perspective, these effects may be mediated through endogenous opioid pathways (*see* PLACEBO for more information). Thus, when considering the putative mechanisms underlying individual differences in pain responses, it is important to recognize that "psychosocial" and "biological" explanations may refer to the same underlying processes described at different levels of analysis. Second, pain is a constructed experience. The central nervous system does not simply "register" the pain signal to produce pain perception, rather the brain constructs the pain experience by integrating a vast array of inputs, including biological factors, current and past psychological events, and sociocultural influences. Most important, all of these factors interact bidirectionally, such that psychosocial factors and interventions can alter biological processes and vice versa. Thus, the ultimate "mosaic" of information that produces the experience of pain is sculpted by these complex interactions. Third, stronger integration of psychological approaches and principles into pain research and treatment will foster much more rapid progress in conceptual, clinical, and scientific endeavors. This principle flows directly from the first two principles. That is, given that mind-body dualism does not work and that psychosocial factors contribute substantially to the constructed pain experience, it logically follows that understanding and successfully treating the experience of pain requires assimilation of these factors.

An interesting issue to ponder is the specific versus nonspecific effects of pain treatment, including psychological therapies. Empirical evidence documents the effectiveness of several forms of psychological treatment for pain in multiple clinical populations. Many of these therapies (e.g., hypnosis, relaxation, cognitive interventions, behavioral therapy, psychodynamic therapy) will likely produce their clinical effects based on some overlapping general mechanisms, but there are also specific effects of some treatments that as yet are not well understood. For example, many psychological therapies may involve nonspecific effects including education, increasing patients' acceptance of pain, instillation of hope, enhanced self-efficacy, and encouraging behavior change, all of which may improve pain-related adjustment. However, specific and direct effects of a given therapy on pain processing (e.g., hypnosis) exist. We need to know more about both the specific and nonspecific effects of psychological treatments for pain.

As the title implies, this is a concise encyclopedia; therefore, an exhaustive review of each topic is beyond the scope of this book. It is my hope that this will provide a broad range of useful information related to pain psychology, and that readers will gain an appreciation for the breadth and depth of psychological contributions to the field of pain management and research. Other books are available for interested readers who wish to obtain more detailed information related to pain psychology. I would recommend the following: *Psychosocial*

Factors in Pain (Gatchel & Turk, 1999); *Psychological Approaches to Pain Management* (Turk & Gatchel, 2002); *Psychosocial Aspects of Pain: A Handbook for Health Care Providers* (Dworkin & Breitbart, 2004); *Pain: Psychological Perspectives* (Hadjistavropoulos & Craig, 2004); and *Psychological Mechanisms of Pain and Analgesia* (Price, 2000).

abuse: Substantial evidence suggests an association between chronic pain and a history of childhood sexual or physical abuse. Rates of self-reported sexual and/or physical abuse history in patients with heterogeneous chronic pain ranged from 28 to 48 percent, often statistically higher than in the general population (Goldberg, 1994; Boisset-Pioro, Esdaile, & Fitzcharles, 1995; Fillingim, Maixner, Sigurdsson, & Kincaid, 1997; Nickel, Egle, & Hardt, 2002; Green, Flowe-Valencia, Rosenblum, & Tait, 1999; Green, Flowe-Valencia, Rosenblum, & Tait, 2001; Toomey, Seville, Mann, Abashian, & Grant, 1995; Wurtele, Kaplan, & Keairnes, 1990). High frequencies of self-reported abuse were also found in specific chronic pain syndromes, including fibromyalgia (Alexander et al., 1998; Boisset-Pioro et al., 1995; Taylor, Trotter, & Csuka, 1995; Walker et al., 1997); gastrointestinal pain (Drossman et al., 1990; Leserman et al., 1996; Scarinci, McDonald-Haile, Bradley, & Richter, 1994); headache (Domino & Haber, 1987); temporomandibular disorders (Fillingim et al., 1997); and pelvic pain (Walker, Katon, Neraas, Jemelka, & Massoth, 1992; Walling et al., 1994). Moreover, self-reported abuse history in patients with chronic pain has been associated with poorer pain-related adjustment (Linton, Larden, & Gillow, 1996; Domino & Haber, 1987; Alexander et al., 1998). In addition to these findings in clinical populations, studies using community-based samples also indicate that a self-reported history of childhood abuse is associated with increased pain-related symptoms (Bendixen, Muus, & Schei, 1994; Fillingim et al., 1997; Fillingim, Wilkinson, & Powell, 1999; Linton, 1997, 2002). In contrast, a recent prospective population-based study examined the association between *documented* childhood abuse and subsequent development of pain (Raphael, Widom, & Lange, 2001). These investigators identified a cohort of 676 adult subjects with court-substantiated cases of abuse or neglect that occurred between 1967 and 1971 before the child reached 11 years old. A control group of 520 subjects was identified that was matched on age, sex, ethnicity, and social class. All participants were interviewed to collect information regarding self-reported history of abuse or neglect as well as psychological and pain-related symptoms. Subjects with documented abuse or neglect history were no more likely to report pain than subjects with no documented abuse history. However, those subjects who retrospectively *reported* a history of abuse or neglect were significantly more likely to report pain compared to those reporting no abuse history. Thus, retrospective recall of abuse history, but not documented abuse, was associated with pain-related symptoms, which highlights the potential limitations of relying solely on self-report to assess both abuse history and pain.

Although the relationship between abuse history and pain-related symptoms is inevitably multiply determined, one possible mechanism explaining the link is that childhood trauma may produce enhanced pain sensitivity. Indeed, several of the pain disorders with high rates of self-reported abuse history are characterized by enhanced sensitivity to experimental pain (Lautenbacher, Rollman, & McCain, 1994; Maixner, Fillingim, Booker, & Sigurdsson, 1995; Verne, Robinson, & Price, 2001; Lautenbacher et al., 1994; Maixner et al., 1995; Verne et al., 2001). Few studies investigated the association between experimental pain responses and abuse history. Evidence of enhanced responses to experimental pain among patients reporting a history of abuse were reported among individuals with gastrointestinal pain (Scarinci et al., 1994) and fibromyalgia (Alexander et al., 1998). However, other investigators reported that abuse history was not related to the pain perception in women with irritable bowel syndrome or in healthy control women (Whitehead et al., 1997), and we reported that abuse history is associated with *decreased* pain sensitivity among patients with orofacial pain (Fillingim et al., 1997) as well as pain-free controls (Fillingim & Edwards, in press). Thus, self-reported abuse history is associated with chronic pain, but the precise nature of the relationship and the underlying mechanisms remain unclear.

acceptance: In recent years, the concept of acceptance of chronic pain has received increasing empirical attention. McCracken (1998) defined acceptance as "acknowledging that one has pain, giving up unproductive attempts to control pain, acting as if pain does not necessarily imply disability, and being able to commit one's efforts toward living a satisfying life despite pain" (p. 22). More recently, three features of acceptance were identified, including (1) acknowledging that a cure for pain is unlikely, (2) shifting one's focus away from pain to nonpain aspects of life, and (3) rejecting the notion that pain reflects personal weakness (Risdon, Eccleston, Crombez, & McCracken, 2003). McCracken reported that higher acceptance was associated with less emotional distress and disability (McCracken, 1998), and accepting pain predicted increased likelihood of patients being classified as adaptive copers (McCracken, Spertus, Janeck, Sinclair, & Wetzel, 1999). More recent findings indicate that acceptance predicts pain-related adjustment (e.g., pain, disability, anxiety, depression) independent of the predictive value of coping (McCracken & Eccleston, 2003; Viane et al., 2003). Thus, interventions to enhance acceptance of pain among patients may produce improved treatment outcomes.

acute pain: Acute pain generally refers to pain lasting less than three months, and it is often mistakenly excluded from discussions of psychosocial influences on pain. Acute pain is ubiquitous and overwhelming evidence indicates that psychological factors exert important influences on acute pain (Williams, 2004). For example, anxiety predicts greater pain following surgery and other procedures, and preoperative anxiety is a consistent predictor of postoperative analgesic consumption (Caumo et al., 2002; Gil, Ginsberg, Muir, Sykes, & Williams, 1990; Nelson, Zimmerman, Barnason, Nieveen, & Schmaderer, 1998; Perry, Parker, White, & Clifford, 1994). Other psychological variables, including cognitive factors, expectancies, social learning, appraisal, and coping, also influence the experience of acute pain (Bandura, Cioffi, Taylor, & Brouillard, 1988; France, France, al'Absi, Ring, & McIntyre, 2002; Pollo et al., 2001). Psychological interventions such as relaxation, distraction, and hypnosis are effective methods for reducing acute pain (Luebbert, Dahme, & Hasenbring, 2001; Montgomery, David, Winkel, Silverstein, & Bovbjerg, 2002; Patterson & Jensen, 2003; Villemure & Bushnell, 2002).

addiction: Addiction is defined as a primary, chronic, neurobiologic disease, with genetic, psychosocial, and environmental factors influencing its development and manifestations (Savage et al., 2003). It is characterized by behaviors that include one or more of the following: impaired control over drug use, compulsive use, continued use despite harm, and craving. Some professionals prefer the terminology from the *Diagnostic and Statistical Manual* (Fourth Edition) of the American Psychiatric Association (DSM-IV), substance dependence. *Substance dependence* is defined as a maladaptive pattern of substance use leading to clinically significant impairment or distress, as manifested by symptoms such as: tolerance, withdrawal, using increasing amounts of the substance, unsuccessful efforts to reduce use, extraordinary efforts to obtain the substance, and use despite harm (American Psychiatric Association, 1994).

Concerns about addiction emerge in virtually any discussion of long-term opioids for chronic pain. Indeed, both patients and physicians report significant concerns about addiction (Gilron, Bailey, Weaver, & Houlden, 2002; Morley-Forster, Clark, Speechley, & Moulin, 2003; Potter et al., 2001). Estimates of the prevalence of addiction among patients with chronic pain vary widely, ranging from 3 to 19 percent (Fishbain, Rosomoff, & Rosomoff, 1992). Some disagreement exists as to whether opioid abuse is increasing. The College on Problems of Drug Dependence task force on prescription opioid nonmedical use and abuse reported that nonmedical use of opioids increased dramatically in the past 10 to 15 years (Zacny et al., 2003). Regarding opioid abuse in proportion to legitimate use, a retrospective analysis of trends in opioid therapy revealed that the medical use of opioids increased dramatically from 1990 to 1996, while evidence of opioid abuse increased only slightly and actually decreased relative to abuse of other substances (Joranson, Ryan, Gilson, & Dahl, 2000). In contrast, Zacny and colleagues (2003) analyzed similar data over a more recent time period (1994-2001) and reported that the ratio of illicit to licit (appropriate) use has increased significantly over that time period, especially for hydromorphone and oxycodone (in 2000 and 2001). Thus, on a population basis, nonmedical use and abuse of opioids has increased substantially in recent years, and it appears that the rate of increase in nonmedical use/abuse has been greater than the increase in legitimate use.

One complicating issue in identifying addiction among patients with chronic pain is the overlap between signs of abuse and common patterns of medication use for pain control in this population. For example, patients with chronic pain may find it necessary to increase their doses over time, they exhibit tolerance and withdrawal symptoms, and they often expend considerable effort to obtain the substance. Rather than representing signs of substance dependence, these symptoms may reflect what has been termed *pseudoaddiction*. This term, originally proposed by Weissman and Haddox (1989), refers to patient behaviors resulting from inadequate analgesia that mimic addiction and resolve with effective pain relief. Although many experts believe that the risk of addiction to prescription opiates is quite low in this population (e.g., Passik & Weinreb, 2000; Portenoy, 1996), prescribers and patients remain quite concerned about the specter of addiction (Moulin, Clark, Speechley, & Morley-Forster, 2002; Gilron & Bailey, 2003; Weiner & Rudy, 2002; Potter et al., 2001; Bendtsen, Hensing, Ebeling, & Schedin, 1999). An often-stated position is that chronic opioids can be safe and effective, with minimal risk of addiction, in carefully selected patients. However, the criteria for this "careful selection" remain unclear. For example, considerable debate exists as to the appropriateness of opioid therapy in patients with a history of substance abuse (Compton & Athanasos, 2003). Additional research is needed to determine the prevalence and predictors of addiction within the chronic pain population and to develop strategies for preventing and treating these problems when they arise.

aging: Several literature reviews suggest that persistent pain may be highly prevalent and disabling during the later years of life (Gagliese & Melzack, 1997a; Gibson & Helme, 2001; Gibson, Katz, Corran, Farrell, & Helme, 1994; Helme & Gibson, 2001; Verhaak, Kerssens, Dekker, Sorbi, & Bensing, 1998). In a recent survey regarding chronic pain in primary care settings, age greater than 40 was a significant predictor of both the onset of a persistent pain condition, and this age group was also more likely not to recover from pain during the 12-month follow-up period (Gureje, Simon, & Von Korff, 2001). It has also been reported that greater expectations of pain, more pain sites, and greater interference of pain with daily activities may occur with aging (Gagliese & Melzack, 1997; Gibson et al., 1994; Harkins, 1996; Harkins & Scott, 1996). Pain in the elderly can adversely impact quality of life and is associated with increased physical disability and mortality (Kendig, Browning, & Young, 2000; Scudds & Robertson, 1998). Although increased disease activity (e.g., osteoarthritis) may contribute to these age-associated increases in the prevalence and impact of pain, age-related alterations in pain perception could also be important.

In a recent review article, Gibson & Helme (2001) note that considerable evidence suggests global age-associated decrements in most perceptual systems, changes in pain perception with aging are not well characterized. In general, elderly adults show a slightly elevated pain threshold and somewhat larger decreases in pain tolerance relative to younger adults (Gibson & Helme, 2001). The effects of age on pain sensitivity likely depend on the characteristics of the painful stimulus. Specifically, older adults exhibit enhanced responsiveness to deeper (Edwards & Fillingim, 2001a), more tonic (Walsh, Schoenfeld, Ramamurthy, & Hoffman, 1989), more intense (Harkins & Chapman, 1977), and more temporally dynamic (Edwards & Fillingim, 2001b) noxious stimuli. One explanation of pattern of results is that aging may be associated with decreased effectiveness of endogenous pain inhibitory systems (Gibson & Helme, 2001; Washington, Gibson, & Helme, 2000). For example, repeated immersion of the hand in cold water produced greater increases in electrical pain thresholds among younger versus older adults (Washington, Gibson, & Helme, 2000), and a similar study reported that repeated cold water pain reduced ratings of heat pain at a remote site (i.e., diffuse noxious inhibitory controls—DNIC) more in younger compared to older adults (Edwards, Fillingim, & Ness, 2003). Thus, aging is associated with increases in clinical pain, which may be due in part to diminished pain inhibition.

alexithymia: Alexithymia refers to a deficit in an individual's ability either to recognize or to express emotions, and patients with chronic pain may score higher on measures of alexithymia than healthy controls (Lumley, Stettner, & Wehmer, 1996; Lumley, Smith, & Longo, 2002; Porcelli, Taylor, Bagby, & De Carne, 1999). The most commonly used measure of alexithymia is the Toronto Alexithymia Scale (Bagby, Taylor, & Parker, 1994; Bagby, Parker, & Taylor, 1994; Taylor, Ryan, & Bagby, 1985; Taylor, Bagby, & Parker, 2003; Parker, Taylor, & Bagby, 2003). Lumley and colleagues (1996) proposed a model whereby alexithymia can influence physical illness. Specifically, they note that alexithymia can affect disease processes directly via its influence on physiological processes (e.g., increased physiological arousal) and behavior (e.g., smoking, poor nutrition, sedentary lifestyle). Moreover, alexithymia can affect illness behavior through its adverse impact on cognition (e.g., appraisal of somatic symptoms, negative affect) and social functioning (e.g., low social support).

allodynia: Allodynia refers to an alteration in pain perception such that normally nonpainful stimuli are perceived as painful (Merskey

& Bogduk, 1994). This phenomenon is often observed in patients with neuropathic pain or complex regional pain syndrome, but is also characteristic of inflammatory pain and other causes of skin sensitization (e.g., sunburn). It is important to note that allodynia is a perceptual phenomenon and can be due to peripheral and/or central sensitization. Historically, before the neurobiology of peripheral and central sensitization was elucidated, allodynia was often mistakenly considered a sign of psychogenic pain.

alternative medicine: As with many other clinical conditions, the use of complementary and alternative medicine (CAM) treatments for pain management has increased dramatically in recent years (Cauffield, 2000; Astin, 1998). One of the difficulties in providing an overview of this topic is the vast array of treatment modalities encompassed by the term CAM, including physical modalities (e.g., acupuncture, massage, chiropractic), herbal medicine, spiritual and faith-based approaches, and nonlocal healing (e.g., prayer). Moreover, consensus is lacking on which therapies should be considered alternative medicine. It is also likely that the efficacy of different CAM therapies will vary across pain conditions, making general conclusions impossible. In general, most reviews of CAM treatment for pain conclude that rigorous scientific evidence supporting the efficacy of many CAM treatments is lacking; however, trends suggestive of benefit do exist (Soeken, 2004; Snyder & Wieland, 2003; Weintraub, 2003; Smith, Collins, Cyna, & Crowther, 2003). Thus, a need exists for additional carefully conducted clinical trials to determine the effectiveness of CAM treatments for pain.

analgesia: The definition of analgesia is "absence of pain in response to stimulation that would normally be painful" (Merskey & Bogduk, 1994, p. 211). The term is often more loosely applied to refer to the reduction in pain elicited by an intervention. Analgesic responses to medications vary widely across individuals and are influenced by multiple psychosocial factors (Price, 2000). In addition, psychological interventions can produce significant analgesic responses, as discussed elsewhere in this book. (*See also* COGNITIVE-BEHAVIORAL THERAPY; HYPNOSIS; PLACEBO.)

anger: Anger is a negative emotion, typically elicited by a perceived wrong, and considerable research indicates that anger is associated with pain. In a recent review of this topic, four important anger constructs were discussed: anger, hostility, aggression, and anger-management style (Greenwood, Thurston, Rumble, Waters, & Keefe, 2003). Anger is typically viewed as a transient state, while hostility refers to an enduring tendency to interpret others' behavior as malicious and aggressive. Hostile individuals often experience anger in a variety of conditions, are likely to be aggressive, and often possess traits of cynicism and distrust. Aggression refers to the behavioral component of anger, including overt or covert destructive and harmful physical or verbal actions aimed at other persons or objects. Anger-management style generally refers to whether individuals externalize or express their anger (i.e., anger out) versus internalizing or inhibiting anger expression (i.e., anger in).

Several lines of evidence support an association of anger with pain responses. First, standardized measures indicate higher levels of anger among patients with chronic pain than in pain-free individuals, and anger is associated with greater pain and higher levels of psychological distress (Fernandez & Turk, 1995; Greenwood et al., 2003). Some evidence suggests that anger may relate to pain in a sex-dependent manner. For example, anger-expression style and hostility were differentially associated with pain in female and male chronic pain patients, such that high hostility with high anger expression predicted the highest pain levels among men, while high hostility with low anger expression predicted the greatest pain among women (Burns, Johnson, Mahoney, Devine, & Pawl, 1996). Burns and colleagues (1998) also found that high anger expression among males was associated with less improvement in lifting capacity following treatment, and high anger suppression was associated with smaller improvements in general activity and depressed mood. These anger variables were not predictive of treatment responses in women.

Anger expression may also relate to pain variables differentially across diagnostic subgroups. For instance, a recent investigation reported that high anger-out scores (i.e., high anger expressiveness) predicted greater pain among patients with upper extremity pain due to complex regional pain syndrome but anger out was associated with lower pain in patients whose upper extremity pain derived from other etiologies (Bruehl, Chung, & Burns, 2003). Similarly, anger out was positively associated with headache activity among patients with migraine but not chronic tension headache (Materazzo, Cathcart, & Pritchard, 2000).

A few studies examined the effects of anger on experimental pain perception. Janssen and colleagues (2001) reported that a laboratory anger induction produced increased tolerance for cold pressor pain; however, higher anger ratings were associated with greater reported pain. More recently, Burns and colleagues (2003) found that high anger-out scores were associated with a higher pain threshold only when preceded by an anger induction task, but not after sadness or joy inductions. High anger-in (i.e., anger suppression) scores were associated with higher levels of reported pain across all emotion inductions. These findings illustrate the complexity of the association between anger and pain responses.

anterior cingulate: The anterior cingulate cortex is a brain region involved in many important functions, including cognition, affect, and pain perception, and altered function of the anterior cingulate is thought to contribute to psychiatric and addictive disorders (Phillips, Drevets, Rauch, & Lane, 2003; Rauch, 2003; Nutt, Lingford-Hughes, & Daglish, 2003; Franken, 2003; Hart, Wade, & Martelli, 2003). Numerous studies of experimental pain demonstrate that the anterior cingulate is activated by noxious stimuli (Casey & Bushnell, 2000; Peyron, Laurent, & Garcia-Larrea, 2000), and some evidence suggests a specific role for the anterior cingulate in processing the affective component of pain (i.e., pain unpleasantness) (Rainville, 2002; Rainville, Duncan, Price, Carrier, & Bushnell, 1997). Thus, this neural structure may represent an important link between psychological processes and the experience of pain.

antidepressants: Antidepressants have been used in the management of chronic pain for decades. Recent meta-analytic reviews demonstrate that antidepressants are more effective than placebo in the management of general chronic pain (Onghena & Van Houdenhove, 1992) as well as low back pain (Salerno, Browning, & Jackson, 2002); fibromyalgia (O'Malley et al., 2000); headache (Tomkins, Jackson, O'Malley, Balden, & Santoro, 2001); neuropathic pain (McQuay, 2002; McQuay et al., 1996); gastrointestinal disorders (Jackson et al., 2000); and somatoform pain (Fishbain, Cutler, Rosomoff, & Rosomoff, 1998). The pain-relieving effects of antidepressants may be independent of their effects on depression; however, insufficient data are available to draw conclusions in most studies (e.g., Jackson et al., 2000; O'Malley et al., 2000; Tomkins, Jackson, O'Malley, Balden, & Santoro, 2001).

The two major classes of antidepressants most frequently used for treating pain, tricyclic antidepressants (TCAs) and selective serotonin reuptake inhibitors (SSRIs), are thought to produce their pain-relieving effects via their pharmacologic actions that augment the functioning of central nervous system serotonergic and noradrenergic pathways, as both of these systems are important in descending pain modulation (Rao, 2002). However, TCAs also produce antagonism at histamine, cholinergic, and NMDA (N-methyl-D-aspartate) receptors and can block ion channels, which may contribute to their analgesic as well as their adverse effects (Rao, 2002). Newer antidepressants (e.g., venlafaxine) block the reuptake of both serotonin and norepinephrine, which may provide more robust analgesic effects. However, no evidence to date supports greater efficacy of one class of antidepressants over another for treating chronic pain.

Several studies investigated the effects of antidepressants on pain perception assessed via laboratory procedures. In a single-dose study of pain in response to electrical stimuli, three antidepressants (desipramine, fluvoxamine, and moclobemide) increased the perceptual pain threshold, and desipramine and moclobemide also increased the R-III nociceptive flexion reflex (Coquoz, Porchet, & Dayer, 1993). Another experiment demonstrated that imipramine elevated the threshold for pain induced by balloon distention of the esophagus in healthy volunteers (Peghini, Katz, & Castell, 1998). Similarly, Enggaard, Poulsen, and colleagues (Poulsen, 2001) found that imipramine reduced perception of electrical pain and also attenuated temporal summation of electrical pain; however, no effects on cold-pressor pain responses were noted. These investigators reported similar effects of venlafaxine; increases in electrical pain tolerance and decreases in temporal summation of electrical pain but no changes in perception of mechanical or cold-pressor pain (Enggaard, Klitgaard, Gram, Arendt-Nielsen, & Sindrup, 2001). In contrast, a 14-day trial of desipramine produced no changes in pain responses to intradermal capsaicin injection (Wallace, Barger, & Schulteis, 2002). Thus, the analgesic effects of antidepressants on experimental pain perception appear to depend on the pain assay.

anxiety: Associations between pain and anxiety have been widely investigated. High levels of anxiety are more prevalent in chronic pain patients than in the general population. For example, a recent community-based study reported that the prevalence of any anxiety disorder in the past year was 35 percent among individuals with arthritis compared to 18 percent in the general population (McWilliams, Cox, & Enns, 2003). Numerous studies also found patients with chronic pain routinely score higher than published norms on psychometric instruments assessing anxiety (Fillingim, Maixner, Kincaid, Sigurdsson, & Harris, 1996; Robinson & Riley, 1999). Moreover, anxiety has been associated with pain severity and other measures of pain-related adjustment in chronic pain patients (McCracken, Spertus, Janeck, Sinclair, & Wetzel, 1999; McCracken & Gross, 1993; McCracken, Gross, & Eccleston, 2002; McCracken, Gross, Aikens, & Carnrike Jr., 1996).

Anxiety has also been consistently associated with acute pain. For example, presurgical anxiety predicts pain and analgesic use following surgery (Croog, Baume, & Nalbandian, 1995; Gil, Ginsberg, Muir, Sykes, & Williams, 1990; Kain, Sevarino, Alexander, Pincus, & Mayes, 2000; Nelson, Zimmerman, Barnason, Nieveen, & Schmaderer, 1998; Perry, Parker, White, & Clifford, 1994). Also, anxiety has been positively correlated with sensitivity to experimentally induced pain in multiple studies (Graffenried, Adler, Abt, Nuesch, & Spiegel, 1978; Rhudy & Meagher, 2000; Robin, Vinard, Vernet Maury, & Saumet, 1987).

The relationship of pain with anxiety may be sex-dependent. For example, higher levels of anxiety were associated with increased experimental pain sensitivity in men but not women (Fillingim, Keefe, Light, Booker, & Maixner, 1996). Similar findings emerged in a recent study of cold-pressor pain, in which high levels of trait anxiety were associated with greater pain sensitivity in males but not females (Jones, Zachariae, & Arendt-Nielsen, 2003). Also, among chronic pain patients, males with high levels of pain-related anxiety reported greater pain severity and poorer pain-related adjustment than males with low levels of anxiety; however, no such association between anxiety and pain symptoms was present for females (Edwards, Augustson, & Fillingim, 2000). Similar findings were reported (McCracken & Houle, 2000; Riley III, Robinson, Wade, Myers, & Price, 2001), and it was recently discovered that pretreatment anxiety was differentially associated with pain treatment outcome among men and women with chronic pain (Edwards, Augustson, & Fillingim, 2003). Specifically, higher anxiety significantly predicted greater pain reductions from treatment among men, but not women.

Thus, anxiety is associated with both acute and chronic pain, and the pain-anxiety relationship may be stronger for men than women.

anxiety sensitivity: Anxiety sensitivity is a construct related to anxiety. However, anxiety sensitivity (AS) refers to the fear of the physiological and emotional signs and symptoms of anxiety, due to concerns that these anxiety symptoms will produce negative consequences (Asmundson, Wright, Norton, & Veloso, 2001). Anxiety sensitivity is typically measured using the Anxiety Sensitivity Index (Reiss, Peterson, Gursky, & McNally, 1986). This construct may be important in the context of pain, as many of the signs and symptoms of anxiety occur naturally in the context of chronic pain. Indeed, AS has been implicated in several chronic pain conditions (Norton, Norton, Asmundson, Thompson, & Larsen, 1999; Asmundson, Norton, & Veloso, 1999; Asmundson, Norton, & Norton, 1999), and measures of AS correlate significantly with measures of fear of pain (Muris, Vlaeyen, & Meesters, 2001; Asmundson et al., 1999). Moreover, in healthy subjects, higher AS was associated with lower pain threshold and higher pain ratings of cold-pressor pain (Keogh & Cochrane, 2002; Keogh & Mansoor, 2001), and a recent study found that caffeine reduced pain perception among women with low AS but not those with high AS (Keogh & Chaloner, 2002).

 Beck Depression Inventory: The Beck Depression Inventory (BDI) is a 21-item self-report measure that assesses both somatic and cognitive/affective symptoms of depression. The BDI shows excellent reliability and validity as an index of depression (Beck et al., 1988) and has been widely used in chronic pain populations (Skevington, Carse, & Williams, 2001; Dworkin et al., 2002; Lebovits, 2000; Wesley, Gatchel, Garofalo, & Polatin, 1999; Holzberg, Robinson, Geisser, & Gremillion, 1996). It is important to recognize that chronic pain patients often endorse somatic symptoms assessed by the BDI, which may artificially inflate their scores. Indeed, several factor-analytic studies of the BDI in chronic pain populations found that the somatic/physical symptoms constitute a separate subscale than the cognitive/affective symptoms of depression (Morley, Williams, & Black, 2002; Williams & Richardson, 1993; Wesley et al., 1999). Moreover, higher cutoff scores for diagnosing clinical depression were proposed for chronic pain patients (Geisser, Roth, & Robinson, 1997).

behavioral factors: The most influential publication concerning the role of behavioral factors in the expression of pain was the book *Behavioral Methods for Chronic Pain and Illness* by Wilbert E. Fordyce (1976). This book discusses the principles of operant conditioning as they relate to the expression of pain behavior and the application of behavioral principles in the treatment of chronic pain. In essence, pain behaviors, as with any other behavior, can be influenced by environmental contingencies, including reinforcement, extinction, and punishment. Pain behaviors (e.g., limping, complaining, grimacing) will increase in frequency when reinforced and will decrease when extinguished (i.e., ignored) or punished. Examples of potential reinforcers are discussed in subsequent sections of this book (e.g., "spousal responses" or "workers' compensation").

Fordyce's book started a revolution in pain treatment during which behaviorally based multidisciplinary pain programs flourished. Early outcome studies of behavioral management for chronic pain produced promising results (Roberts & Reinhardt, 1980; Guck, Skultety, Meilman, & Dowd, 1985). Also growing out of Fordyce's work was the development of a systematic approach to assessing pain behavior. Keefe and colleagues developed and validated methodology for quantifying overt pain behaviors (e.g., bracing, guarding, grimacing, rubbing, and sighing) in patients with chronic pain (Keefe, Wilkins, & Cook, 1984; Keefe & Hill, 1985; Keefe, Crisson, Maltie, Bradley, & Gil, 1986; Keefe & Dolan, 1986).

Another important component of behavioral models in chronic pain is that of classical (i.e., Pavlovian) conditioning. Classical conditioning occurs when a previously neutral stimulus (the conditioned stimulus—CS) or cue acquires the ability to elicit a response as a result of being paired with a stimulus (the unconditioned stimulus—US) that naturally elicits that response. For example, after an acute back injury, walking (the CS) may be painful (the US) and the patient may exhibit a limp due to the pain. Over time, through being paired with pain, walking can acquire the ability to elicit the limp even when pain has subsided. An important component of treatment to remedy this conditioning is exposure therapy such that the conditioned association between walking and limping will be extinguished. Such principles were applied to address fear avoidance in patients with chronic low back pain (e.g., Vlaeyen, de Jong, Geilen, Heuts, & van Breukelen, 2002).

In addition to their clinical relevance, operant and classical conditioning were examined in laboratory studies. For example, Flor, Birmbaumer, Schulz, Grusser, & Mucha (2002) demonstrated that stress-induced analgesia can be classically conditioned in humans. Also, numerous investigators reported that classical conditioning contributes to opioid tolerance and some forms of hyperalgesia. Operant conditioning of pain responses has also been demonstrated in humans. Specifically, Flor, Knost, & Birbaumer (2002) provided positive feedback to healthy controls and low back pain patients for higher (up-training) versus lower (down-training) ratings of electrical pain stimuli. Pain ratings were increased by up-training and decreased by down-training for both pain patients and healthy controls, and there was evidence that the pain patients' responses were more resistant to extinction. Thus, behavioral factors are broadly important in both acute and chronic pain.

beliefs: Considerable interest exists in patients' beliefs and attitudes about pain, based on the assumption that these beliefs can have important influence on patients' behavioral and psychological response to painful symptoms. Numerous scales to assess pain-related beliefs have been developed over the years, but only the two most widely used instruments will be discussed here. A more comprehensive discussion of the other instruments is available elsewhere (DeGood & Tait, 2001). Williams and Thorn (1989) developed the Pain Beliefs and Perceptions Inventory to assess patients' conceptualizations and interpretations of pain. The instrument was designed to assess three dimensions of pain beliefs: self-blame, the mysteriousness of pain, and beliefs about the duration of pain (Williams & Thorn, 1989). However, subsequent studies suggested a four-factor solution, which included these three dimensions plus a factor related to beliefs regarding the permanence of pain (Williams & Keefe, 1991; Herda, Siegeris, & Basler, 1994; Morley & Wilkinson, 1995). Pain beliefs appear to be clinically relevant as they are associated with pain severity, affective distress, and the coping strategies that patients use in several studies (Williams, Robinson, & Geisser, 1994; Williams & Keefe, 1991; Herda et al., 1994).

The Survey of Pain Attitudes (SOPA) is now in its third revision and the full version includes 57 items and assesses seven dimensions of patients' beliefs regarding pain: control, disability, medical cures, solicitude, medication, emotion, and harm (Jensen, Turner, & Romano, 2000; Jensen, Turner, Romano, & Lawler, 1994; Jensen, Karoly, & Huger, 1987). Two shortened versions are also available (Jensen et al., 2000; Tait & Chibnall, 1997). Multiple studies demonstrate that the SOPA has adequate psychometric properties (DeGood & Tait, 2001). Moreover, pain beliefs assessed via the SOPA predict pain-related adjustment and treatment-induced changes in beliefs are associated with treatment responses (Jensen et al., 2001; Jensen & Karoly, 1992; Jensen, Romano, Turner, Good, & Wald, 1999; Tait & Chibnall, 1998). Thus, pain beliefs can be systematically assessed and are clinically important.

biofeedback: Biofeedback (BFB) refers to a group of treatments in which physiological monitoring equipment is used to provide the patient with real-time information regarding specific symptom-related biological responses (e.g., muscle activity, blood flow, skin temperature). Therapeutic efforts are then directed at enabling the patient to control these physiological responses, thereby improving his or her symptoms. One of the most common applications of biofeedback has been in the treatment of chronic headache, in which the goal is to reduce muscle activity in the muscles of the forehead or increase peripheral skin temperature. Combined results from several meta-analyses suggest that biofeedback produces a clinically significant improvement in approximately 40 to 50 percent of tension-type or migraine headache patients, effects comparable to pharmacotherapy. Biofeedback also seems to be effective in the management of temporomandibular disorders with results that are comparable to intraoral appliances, a standard conservative treatment (Myers, White, & Heft, 2002; Turk, Zaki, & Rudy, 1993). Some evidence also supports the effectiveness of BFB for low back pain (Newton-John, Spence, & Schotte, 1995; Nielson & Weir, 2001), though some studies do not (Bush, Ditto, & Feuerstein, 1985). Typically, rather than serving as a stand-alone intervention, BFB is provided as part of a multicomponent treatment program for chronic pain, and the unique contribution of BFB to clinical improvement in this scenario is difficult to discern.

Several possible mechanisms of action have been proposed to explain the clinical effects of biofeedback. The Operant Model posits that BFB reinforces patients for producing the appropriate symptom-reducing response. The Motor Skills Model suggests that BFB enhances specific physiological or motor skills that assist in pain control. Systems theory holds that biofeedback serves as a negative feedback loop to promote homeostasis. Another model is that BFB works by assisting the patient in producing the general relaxation response. The Awareness Model proposes that BFB enhances awareness of interoceptive cues, which the patient can use to control their pain. Finally, according to the Cognitive Model, thoughts mediate the relationship between the environment and physiological responses to the environment and BFB helps patients reduce their pain by altering their thoughts. In considering the mechanism(s) underlying BFB's effects, a previous study of BFB for headache is worth noting. Patients underwent forehead EMG (electromyographic) BFB and were provided either high or moderate bogus-success feedback, and half of the patients were unwittingly being trained to *increase* their forehead muscle tension while the other half were trained to decrease tension (Holroyd et al., 1984). The results indicated that patients in the high- success feedback group improved significantly more than the low- success group, regardless of whether they increased or decreased their muscle tension. This result suggests that cognitive factors may be particularly important. Regardless of mechanisms, BFB appears to be a beneficial treatment for many chronic pain conditions, especially when combined with other treatment approaches.

biopsychosocial model: The biopsychosocial model of pain posits that the experience of and response to pain is determined by complex and dynamic interactions among biological, psychological, and socio-cultural factors (Turk, 1996). This model is an answer to the inadequacy of the disease model, which insists on a high correspondence between pain and pathology. The literature is replete with evidence that pain and tissue damage are poorly correlated, that tremendous interindividual differences exist in the perception of pain, and that pain-related symptoms such as emotional distress, disability, and other indices of suffering cannot be predicted from pathophysiology. The biopsychosocial model is represented graphically as follows.

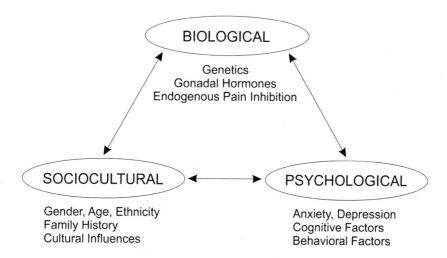

cancer pain: A large proportion of patients with cancer experience clinically significant pain. Pain occurs in up to 50 percent of patients undergoing active treatment for a solid tumor and as many as 90 percent of those with advanced disease (Portenoy et al., 1994; Cleeland et al., 1994). The prevalence of pain varies with the site, type, and stage of cancer as well as the treatment regimen. For example, up to 80 percent of patients with metastatic cancer experience pain, and pain also is highly prevalent for gynecologic, prostate, and head and neck cancers (Anderson, Syrjala, & Cleeland, 2001). Multiple etiologies contribute to pain in cancer, including treatment-induced pain and pain caused by the disease process, and pain can be nociceptive and/or neuropathic (Breitbart & Payne, 2004; Anderson et al., 2001). In addition to its adverse effects on quality of life, non-human animal studies demonstrate that uncontrolled pain can promote tumor growth (Page, Blakely, & Ben Eliyahu, 2001), and pain may predict poorer survival (Herndon et al., 1999). Moreover, breakthrough pain is associated with increased health care costs (Fortner, Okon, & Portenoy, 2002). Although it has been estimated that up to 90 percent of cancer pain can be adequately controlled (World Health Organization, 1996), due to patient-level and system-level barriers, cancer pain continues to be poorly managed (Anderson et al., 2001).

As with other forms of pain, psychosocial variables are associated with cancer pain. A recent literature review revealed strong evidence that psychological distress is associated with cancer pain and moderate evidence that pain is associated with low social support (Zaza & Baine, 2002). Also, psychoeducational interventions appear to be effective for reducing pain and pain-related distress among patients with cancer (Devine, 2003). Education of both patients and providers, improved assessment of cancer pain, and optimal implementation of available medical and nonpharmacological treatments are needed to enhance pain management in persons with cancer.

catastrophizing: Simply defined, catastrophizing refers to a negative cognitive response to experienced or anticipated pain in which the individual attends selectively to and/or magnifies the aversive aspects of the painful situation. Sullivan and colleagues developed the Pain Catastrophizing Scale (PCS), which assesses three dimensions of catastrophizing: magnification, rumination, and helplessness (Sullivan, Bishop, & Pivik, 1995). Sample items include: "It's terrible and I think it's never going to get any better" and "I can't seem to get it out of my mind." The Coping Strategies Questionnaire includes a seven-item subscale that assesses catastrophizing (e.g., "It's awful and I feel that it overwhelms me," "I worry all the time about whether it will end") (Rosenstiel & Keefe, 1983).

Considerable discussion exists regarding the theoretical conceptualization of catastrophizing. For example, is catastrophizing a coping strategy, a product of negative affectivity, a cognitive appraisal process, or an attentional set (Sullivan et al., 2001)? The communal coping model of catastrophizing proposes that catastrophizing is a coping response designed to attain interpersonal goals (e.g., eliciting support) and its negative impact on pain is an unfortunate coincidence (Thorn, Ward, Sullivan, & Boothby, 2003).

Regardless of these conceptual issues, an abundant and growing literature reveals the clinical importance of catastrophizing in both acute and chronic pain. Measures of catastrophizing have been associated with increased pain severity, higher levels of emotional distress, and greater disability among patients with chronic pain (Sullivan et al., 2001). Catastrophizing has also been associated with enhanced sensitivity to experimentally induced pain (France, France, al'Absi, Ring, & McIntyre, 2002; Geisser, Robinson, & Pickren,

1992), as well as greater pain during medical/dental procedures (Sullivan et al., 2001). Recent evidence suggests that reductions in catastrophizing predict better outcomes from multidisciplinary treatment for chronic pain (Burns, Kubilus, Bruehl, Harden, & Lofland, 2003). Moreover, some group differences in catastrophizing were reported, with women reporting greater catastrophizing than men (Fillingim, Wilkinson, & Powell, 1999; Keefe et al., 2000; Osman et al., 2000) and African Americans reporting greater catastrophizing than whites (Campbell, Fillingim, & Edwards, 2005). Thus, catastrophizing is a highly clinically relevant construct and research to further elucidate the nature of catastrophizing will be useful.

chest pain: Chest pain is among the most common conditions seen in primary care settings (Kroenke, Arrington, & Mangelsdorff, 1990) and is often classified as cardiac versus noncardiac in origin. Cardiac chest pain, or angina, results from myocardial ischemia due to stenosis of the coronary blood vessels. Angina is associated with diminished quality of life among patients with heart disease (Kiebzak, Pierson, Campbell, & Cook, 2002; Spertus et al., 2002; Brorsson, Bernstein, Brook, & Werko, 2002). Myocardial ischemia is often brought on by physical exertion (e.g., exercise), but can also be elicited by psychological stress. Interestingly, ischemia induced by psychological stress is less likely to be accompanied by pain (i.e., silent ischemia) than exercise-induced ischemia, which could be due to the greater beta-endorphin response to psychological stress (Miller et al., 1993). Psychological factors including anger, anxiety, depression, and stress have all been associated with the frequency of angina (Rumsfeld et al., 2003; Lewin, 1997). Recent evidence suggests that cognitive-behavioral treatment can reduce the frequency of angina (Lewin et al., 2002).

Noncardiac chest pain (NCCP) refers to chest pain not due to cardiovascular disease. NCCP is a heterogeneous diagnosis and refers to pain from multiple sources, including gastroesophageal reflux disease (GERD), esophageal spasm, musculoskeletal pain, and panic disorder (Eslick, Jones, & Talley, 2003). NCCP is quite common, with a prevalence of up to 25 percent (Eslick et al., 2003), and more than 50 percent of patients referred to cardiologists are diagnosed with NCCP (Thurston, Keefe, Bradley, Rama Krishnan, & Caldwell, 2001). Psychological contributions to NCCP have also been reported.

Specifically, anxiety disorders are more frequent among patients with NCCP compared to other chronic pain syndromes (Thurston et al., 2001). Also, patients with NCCP tend to use passive coping strategies and exhibit greater sensitivity to balloon distention of the esophagus compared to healthy controls (Bradley, Richter, Scarinci, Haile, & Schan, 1992). Several studies demonstrated that cognitive-behavioral interventions are effective in terms of pain reduction, improved psychological function, and reduced activity impairments (Thurston et al., 2001).

child abuse: *See* ABUSE.

children: Acute pain is ubiquitous among children, but chronic pain is also far more prevalent in this population than some would expect. This topic is covered thoroughly in McGrath & Finley (2003). Recurrent headache and abdominal pain are among the most common chronic pain conditions among children (McGrath et al., 2000), but juvenile rheumatoid arthritis, fibromyalgia, and other musculoskeletal pains also affect large numbers of children (Anthony & Schanberg, 2001; Malleson & Clinch, 2003). Chronic pain is associated with diminished quality of life in children, and psychological factors (e.g., depression, anxiety, coping) predict pain severity and disability (Merlijn et al., 2003; Hunfeld, Perquin, Bertina, et al., 2002; Kashikar-Zuck, Goldschneider, Powers, Vaught, & Hershey, 2001). Moreover, psychological therapies are effective for treating chronic pain in children, though much of the evidence is limited to headache and recurrent abdominal pain (Eccleston, Morley, Williams, Yorke, & Mastroyannopoulou, 2002; Weydert, Ball, & Davis, 2003). Cognitive-behavioral interventions are also effective in reducing pain and distress in children undergoing medical procedures (Powers, 1999).

Pain in children presents specific challenges not typically present when considering pain in adults. For example, the developmental stage of the child influences pain assessment. Numerous instruments have been developed and validated for assessing pain in children (McGrath & Gillespie, 2001). Particularly difficult is pain measurement in infants. Indeed, pain in infants is routinely undertreated, perhaps due in part to the unavailability of verbal reports of pain (Anand, 2001). However, pain in neonates can be assessed reliably using a combination of behavioral and physiological indices (Morison, Grunau, Oberlander, & Whitfield, 2001; Morison et al., 2003). Recent evidence indicates that early painful experiences can produce long-lasting changes in the central nervous system that render the organism more sensitive to subsequent painful stimuli; therefore, adequate pain management in early childhood is imperative (Porter, Grunau, & Anand, 1999; Ruda, Ling, Hohmann, Peng, & Tachibana, 2000). Many pharmacologic treatments for pain have not been specifically evaluated among children, and their effectiveness, safety, and optimal doses in children are often not known. Also, family dynamics are highly influential in pediatric pain, which must be considered when implementing treatment protocols (Schanberg et al., 2001; Hunfeld, Perquin, Duivenvoorden, et al., 2001; Palermo, 2000).

chronic pain: Chronic pain typically refers to pain lasting six months or longer, though some definitions set the criterion at three months. Chronic pain is highly prevalent, affecting more than 20 percent of the population (Gallagher, 1999). Chronic pain is typically distinguished from acute pain based on temporal characteristics; however, other important differences should be noted. First the inciting stimulus is typically known for acute pain but is often not fully understood in chronic pain. Second, psychological factors are considered to be more strongly associated with chronic than acute pain, though as this book attests, psychological factors are highly relevant to all forms of pain. Third, in contrast to acute pain, chronic pain often no longer serves an adaptive role as a warning signal.

cognitive-behavioral therapy: Cognitive-behavioral therapy (CBT) represents the most commonly used and empirically validated form of psychological treatment for the management of pain. CBT generally refers to a treatment approach that operates based on the assumption that thoughts and environmental events influence the experience of pain and patients' responses to pain. Therefore, interventions to alter thoughts and environmental contingencies (i.e., the antecedents and consequences of pain behaviors) will be effective components of pain management. CBT includes the behavioral concepts discussed previously (*see* BEHAVIORAL FACTORS), but adds the important mediating role of thoughts. The cognitive component of treatment attempts to replace patients' maladaptive thinking patterns (e.g., catastrophizing) with more effective coping thoughts (e.g., improved self-efficacy, acceptance).

Turk and Rudy (1989) identified five assumptions that underlie CBT interventions. First, individuals actively process information regarding internal stimuli and environmental events, and their behaviors are influenced by their expectations as well as their appraisal of the consequences of their behavior. Second, thoughts influence emotional and physiological responses, which can influence behavior, and behavior, emotions and physiological responses can influence thoughts. Third, behaviors are influenced by environmental events, and vice versa. Fourth, in order to be effective, interventions must address the emotional, cognitive and behavioral dimensions of patients' problems. Finally, if patients are to learn effective methods of coping with their pain, then they must become active participants in treatment.

CBT typically includes training in many of the following skills: education, relaxation training, pleasant-activity scheduling, pacing of activities, cognitive restructuring, and distraction. Numerous controlled trials demonstrate the effectiveness of CBT for reducing pain and disability and improving psychological adjustment among patients with chronic pain (Eccleston, Morley, Williams, Yorke, & Mastroyannopoulou, 2002; Morley, Eccleston, & Williams, 1999; van Tulder et al., 2001). Several studies of multidisciplinary treatment that includes a CBT component indicate that cognitive changes occurring during the course of treatment predict outcome. For example, reductions in catastrophizing and increased self-efficacy for controlling pain predict better outcomes from treatment (Burns, Kubilus, Bruehl, Harden, & Lofland, 2003; Jensen, Turner, & Romano, 2001; Jensen, Turner, & Romano, 1994).

complex regional pain syndrome: Complex regional pain syndrome (CRPS) refers to the painful syndromes that were formerly titled reflex sympathetic dystrophy (RSD) and causalgia. RSD was an unsatisfactory term, as many cases of RSD appeared to be sympathetically independent and dystrophy was not always present (Merskey & Bogduk, 1994). CRPS, Type I, is now the term for RSD. The definition of CRPS, Type I, is "a syndrome that usually develops after an initiating noxious event, is not limited to the distribution of a single peripheral nerve, and is apparently disproportionate to the inciting event" (Merskey & Bogduk, p. 41). An extremity is the most likely affected site, and associated features include edema, changes in skin blood flow, and abnormal sudomotor activity. Pain is typically described as burning and allodynia and hyperalgesia are frequently present. CRPS, Type II, refers to what was previously termed causalgia. The definition is "Burning pain, allodynia, and hyperpathia usually in the hand or foot after partial injury of a nerve or one of its major branches" (p. 42). Pain is described as constant and burning and many of the associated features of CRPS, Type I, may also be present.

A recent epidemiologic study suggests that CRPS is relatively rare (20.6 cases per 100,000) and that spontaneous resolution is common (Sandroni et al., 2003); however, these results have been questioned (Bennett & Harden, 2003). Quantitative sensory testing reveals altered pain perception in patients with CRPS (Kemler, Schouten, & Gracely, 2000; Rommel, Malin, Zenz, & Janig, 2001). Some evidence suggests that psychological factors may be important in these patients. For example, CRPS patients report more stressful life events and showed higher levels of psychological distress compared to healthy controls (Geertzen, Dijkstra, Groothoff, ten Duis, & Eisma, 1998; Geertzen, Bruijn-Kofman, de Bruijn, van de Wiel, & Dijkstra, 1998; Rommel et al., 2001). One study investigated whether patients with CRPS, Type I, were more psychologically disturbed than patients with other types of limb pain and patients with low back pain (Bruehl, Husfeldt, Lubenow, Nath, & Ivankovich, 1996). CRPS patients had higher levels of somatization, anxiety, and depression compared to back pain patients, but differed from the other limb pain group only in somatization. A daily diary study of CRPS patients revealed that pain led to increased anger, depression, and anxiety, and that increases in depression contributed to higher pain levels (Feldman, Downey, & Schaffer-Neitz, 1999). More recently, high anger expression was found to predict more pain in CRPS patients but less pain in non–CRPS limb pain patients (Bruehl, Chung, & Burns, 2003). The authors surmised that the sympathetic activation associated with anger expression may have specific effects on the sympathetically related pain of CRPS.

consciousness: The study of consciousness (e.g., philosophical, cognitive, neurophysiological) has many approaches and many models of consciousness exist. In psychology, consciousness is often conceptualized as awareness, especially with regard to sensory experience. Chapman (1999) proposes a model of pain based on a consciousness framework, which incorporates neurobiological and psychosocial contributions but also emphasizes that the experience of pain is ultimately constructed based on internal representations that are driven by three features of consciousness. They are coherence (i.e., organizing elements of awareness into meaningful wholes); sense of self (i.e., a concept of the self as a whole that is in relation to others); and purposiveness (i.e., goal direction and intentionality).

conversion disorder: Conversion disorder refers to a psychiatric disorder in which patients exhibit motor or sensory symptoms that are not intentionally produced and cannot be explained based on medical findings (American Psychiatric Association, 1994). In conversion disorder, psychological factors are thought to be associated with the symptoms. Conversion disorder refers to the same condition that Freud termed hysteria. Historically, conversion disorder referred to the psychoanalytic concept that intrapsychic conflict is "converted" into physical symptoms as a defense mechanism, thereby allowing the individual to avoid the psychological distress associated with the original source of conflict. This avoidance of intrapsychic conflict and the associated distress is the "primary gain" of experiencing the physical symptom. This produces one of the classically reported hallmarks of conversion disorder or hysteria, *la belle indifference* (the grand indifference), which describes the apparent absence of psychological distress displayed by conversion patients despite the presence of physical symptoms that are often disabling and severe. In addition to this primary gain, there may also be "secondary gain," which refers to external benefits that the patient receives due to the symptoms (e.g., monetary compensation, avoidance of responsibility). Conversion disorder appears to be rare in the general population, but may be present in up to 3 percent of mental health clinic patients (American Psychiatric Association, 1994).

coping: Coping refers to the cognitive/affective and behavioral efforts in which persons engage, in response to perceived demands. Pain coping involves individuals' responses to the demands of pain. Although some debate this issue, most investigators maintain that pain coping includes both adaptive and maladaptive responses. The most commonly used instrument to assess pain coping is the Coping

Strategies Questionnaire (CSQ) (Rosenstiel & Keefe, 1983). Originally, this instrument includes 44 items and yields seven subscales each reflecting a different method of coping with pain: diverting attention, reinterpreting pain sensations, ignoring pain sensations, calming self-statements, increasing behavioral activity, catastrophizing, and praying and hoping. Subsequent factor analyses provide general support for most of these subscales, and higher-order factors (e.g., passive versus active coping) have also emerged (Robinson et al., 1997; Swartzman, Gwadry, Shapiro, & Teasell, 1994). Also, patients' responses on the CSQ were related to pain severity and psychological distress, providing evidence of the clinical validity of this coping measure (Robinson et al., 1997; Riley III, Robinson, & Geisser, 1999; Nicassio, Schoenfeld-Smith, Radojevic, & Schuman, 1995). Other measures of pain coping include the Vanderbilt Pain Management Inventory (Brown & Nicassio, 1987) and the Chronic Pain Coping Inventory (Jensen, Turner, Romano, & Strom, 1995). Interestingly, there is stronger evidence that higher levels of maladaptive coping (e.g., catastrophizing) are associated with poorer pain-related adjustment than evidence that adaptive coping is related to better adjustment (Jensen, Turner, Romano, & Karoly, 1991). As previously discussed (*see* COGNITIVE-BEHAVIORAL THERAPY), a central goal of psychological interventions for pain is to enhance patients' coping skills. Improved coping skills are an important predictor of successful treatment outcome (Burns, Kubilus, Bruehl, Harden, & Lofland, 2003; Jensen, Turner, & Romano, 2001; Jensen, Turner, & Romano, 1994; Tota-Faucette, Gil, Williams, Keefe, & Goli, 1993).

Coping is also related to acute pain and experimental pain sensitivity. For example, reported pain coping predicted pain severity and interference of pain with activity in a sample of healthy young adults (Lester, Lefebvre, & Keefe, 1996). Also, catastrophizing predicted the severity of postoperative pain (Jacobsen & Butler, 1996; Tripp, Stanish, Reardon, Coady, & Sullivan, 2003) and is related to enhanced experimental pain sensitivity (France, France, al'Absi, Ring, & McIntyre, 2002; Geisser, Robinson, & Pickren, 1992). In addition, coping interventions can reduce the perception of acute and experimentally induced pain (Bandura, O'Leary, Taylor, Gauthier, & Gossard, 1987; Villemure & Bushnell, 2002), and one study suggested that coping skills training increased pain tolerance in part via an endogenous opioid mechanism (Bandura et al., 1987). Thus, coping is an important determinant of responses to both acute and chronic pain, and training in pain coping skills can significantly alter the experience of pain.

cortisol: Cortisol is a hormone secreted by the adrenal glands. It is frequently used as a physiological marker of the stress response, and may have particular relevance to pain. Specifically, cortisol may be a biochemical marker of poorly controlled pain. For example, cortisol is increased by experimentally applied pain (Greisen et al., 1999; al'Absi, Petersen, & Wittmers, 2002; Zimmer, Basler, Vedder, & Lautenbacher, 2003). Also, some chronic pain conditions are associated with altered cortisol secretion (Crofford, 1998; Jones, Rollman, & Brooke, 1997; Korszun et al., 2002). Abnormalities of cortisol secretion may reflect chronic hypothalamic-pituitary-adrenocortical activation, which may be associated with a proinflammatory neuroimmune response that could lead to enhanced pain responses (Hurwitz & Morgenstern, 2001).

culture: *See* ETHNICITY.

depression: The term *depression* can refer to a specific psychiatric disorder but it is also used to describe subclinical feelings of sadness and diminished enjoyment from life. The diagnostic criteria for major depression include: depressed mood, loss of interest or pleasure in activities, weight change, altered sleep, psychomotor changes, fatigue, feelings of worthlessness or guilt, diminished concentration, and morbid thinking, including suicidal ideation (American Psychiatric Association, 1994). It is notable that many of these symptoms, especially the somatic ones, are characteristic of chronic pain disorder independent of depression, which makes diagnosis of depression among chronic pain patients particularly challenging. In addition to the psychiatric diagnosis, depression is often conceptualized as a continuous variable that can be assessed using psychometric instruments. Examples include the Beck Depression Inventory (Beck & Steer, 1987), the Center for Epidemiological Studies-Depression Scale (Radloff, 1977), and the Zung Self-Rating Depression Scale (Zung, 1965).

Voluminous evidence indicates that the prevalence of major depression is substantially higher among chronic pain patients than in the general population (Dersh, Polatin, & Gatchel, 2002; Egger, Costello, Erkanli, & Angold, 1999; Gatchel, 1996; Hudson, Goldenberg, Pope, Keck, & Schlesinger, 1992; Kight, Gatchel, & Wesley, 1999; Korszun, Hinderstein, & Wong, 1996; Polatin, Kinney, Gatchel, Lillo, & Mayer, 1993). However, as Banks and Kerns (1996) point out, elevated rates of depression occur in many chronic medical conditions; therefore comparisons to other patient populations are needed. These authors state that the available evidence suggests that depression is indeed more common among chronic pain populations than in other chronic medical conditions. The direction of the relationship between chronic pain and depression has been addressed in several studies. For example, Polatin and colleagues (1993) reported that 54 percent of chronic back pain patients who met lifetime diagnostic criteria for major depression developed their depressive disorder before the onset of pain. In another study, depression predated the onset of pain in only 42 percent of patients (Atkinson, Slater, Patterson, Grant, & Garfin, 1991). Breslau, Lipton, Stewart, Schultz, & Welch (2003) and Breslau and colleagues (2000) have shown a bidirectional relationship between major depression and migraine headache, such that each increases risk for the other. Interestingly, the relationship between nonmigraine severe headache and major depression was unidirectional, with headache increasing risk of depression but not vice versa (Breslau et al., 2000). A meta-analysis of the literature on pain and depression, Fishbain, Cutler, Rosomoff, & Rosomoff (1997) found evidence supporting the notion that depression is a consequence rather than an antecedent of pain. In addition to these findings, which used specific diagnostic criteria for major depression, numerous studies reported that chronic pain patients have elevated scores on psychometric instruments that assess the degree of depressive symptomatology (Geisser, Roth, & Robinson, 1997; Holzberg, Robinson, Geisser, & Gremillion, 1996; Robinson & Riley, 1999). Higher levels of depression are associated with greater pain and pain-related disability (Reid, Guo, Towle, Kerns, & Concato, 2002; Haythornthwaite, Sieber, & Kerns, 1991), and depression predicts poorer outcome from surgical interventions for pain (Block, 1999). Although the previous literature focuses on the prevalence of depression among patients known to have chronic pain, it is also important to consider the relationship of depression and pain outside of populations of patients with chronic pain. For example, somatic complaints, including pain, are widespread among depressed individuals even in the absence of any pain-related diagnosis (Greenberg, Leong, Birnbaum, & Robinson, 2003; Briley, 2003). Moreover, community studies indicate a significant association between pain and depression (Katon, 2003; Hotopf, Mayou, Wadsworth, & Wessely, 1998), and depressed patients with chronic pain report more severe psychological distress and greater health care utilization compared to depressed patients who do not have pain (Bao, Sturm, & Croghan, 2003). Also, depression may be associated with alterations in pain perception. For example, depressed patients reported more pain after abdominal surgery than nondepressed patients (Kudoh, Katagai, & Takazawa, 2002). Also, numerous studies examined experimental pain perception in depressed versus nondepressed patients. A review of the literature indicated that most studies of pain perception in depressed patients reveal that depression is associated with decreased sensitivity to experimentally induced pain (Lautenbacher & Krieg, 1994). However, subsequent findings indicate that depressed patients show lower tolerance for ischemic arm pain, a more tonic and clinically relevant experimental pain stimulus (Pinerua-Shuhaibar et al., 1999). Thus, it is possible that depression is associated with decreased sensitivity to brief, superficial pain but enhanced sensitivity to tonic, clinically relevant pain, perhaps due to altered endogenous pain modulation. It is also interesting that experimentally induced sadness is associated with lower pain tolerance (Willoughby, Hailey, Mulkana, & Rowe, 2002).

The reasons for the high comorbidity between pain and depression are the topic of considerable discussion. Historically, some investigators suggested that chronic pain was a variant of depression (Blumer & Heilbronn, 1982; Ward et al., 1982), however this explanation seems unlikely to account for most cases given that the typical temporal pattern for the association is that chronic pain predates depression. Several psychological models explaining the link between pain and depression have been described, including the cognitive-distortion model, the behavioral model, the learned-helplessness model, and the diathesis-stress model (Banks & Kerns, 1996). In addition, biological mechanisms may be important, since both pain and depression are heavily influenced by similar neuroendocrine and neurotransmitter systems (Campbell, Clauw, & Keefe, 2003). Inevitably, both psychosocial and biological factors contribute to the association of depression and pain.

diathesis-stress model: The diathesis-stress model has been applied to explain the development of complex, multidetermined medical and psychiatric conditions. The diathesis refers to an organismic trait that confers an increased tendency or risk to develop a given disorder, which typically is conceptualized as a genetic predisposition but could also refer to psychological characteristics. The stress component refers to some experienced life event that activates the diathesis leading to the emergence of the disorder. This model applies well to the development of chronic pain. For example, Banks and Kerns (1996) proposed a diathesis-stress framework to explain the development of depression after the onset of chronic pain. They suggest that chronic pain serves as the stressor and it interacts with preexisting characteristics (e.g., limited coping resources, personality characteristics) to produce depression. The diathesis-stress model can also be applied to the development of chronic pain itself (Dworkin & Banks, 1999). Specifically, multiple neurobiological (e.g., genetic factors, pain history) and psychosocial (personality traits, childhood trauma, psychopathology) may represent risk factors for the development of chronic pain, and these diatheses can be activated by a stressor (e.g., illness, injury, or other major life events).

disability: Disability represents an important symptom dimension among individuals with chronic pain. Disability refers to "an inability to carry out necessary tasks in any important domain of life due to a medical condition" (Robinson, 2001, p. 249). It is important to recognize that disability is determined by factors other than disease severity and pain intensity, including psychosocial variables such as coping, emotional distress, self-efficacy and expectancies (Arnstein, Caudill, Mandle, Norris, & Beasley, 1999; Arnstein, 2000; Ciccone & Just, 2001; Evers, Kraaimaat, Geenen, Jacobs, & Bijlsma, 2003; French et al., 2000; Rejeski, Miller, Foy, Messier, & Rapp, 2001). Disability evaluation is often conducted in chronic pain patients for medicolegal reasons; however, in its more generic sense the term disability is used to denote the impact of pain on a patient's occupational and social functioning. It can be assessed through tests of functional capacity and/or through self-report instruments on which patients report their level of disability. The Oswestry Disability Index (Fairbank & Pynsent, 2000; Fairbank, Couper, Davies, & O'Brien, 1980) and the Roland-Morris Disability Questionnaire (Roland & Morris, 1983a, 1983b) are two commonly used self-report instruments. Self-report and physical performance measures of function are only modestly correlated, and it has been suggested that using both types of assessment is optimal (Lee, Simmonds, Novy, & Jones, 2001; Simmonds et al., 1998). Psychological factors are important predictors of disability in chronic pain patients. For example, even after controlling for pain severity and duration, depression, and somatization, patients' expectancies that work activities would increase their pain and injury were significant predictors of work disability (Ciccone & Just, 2001). Moreover, psychological distress, self-efficacy, and pain beliefs are independent predictors of disability in chronic pain (Barry, Guo, Kerns, Duong, & Reid, 2003; Reid, Guo, Towle, Kerns, & Concato, 2002; Ciccone & Just, 2001; Walsh & Radcliffe, 2002; Mannion et al., 2001).

distraction: Distraction is an important strategy in cognitively coping with pain. Numerous studies demonstrate that distraction interventions significantly reduce perceptual responses to acute clinical and experimental pain (Hoffman, Patterson, Carrougher, & Sharar, 2001; Hoffman, Patterson, & Carrougher, 2000; Johnson, Breakwell, Douglas, & Humphries, 1998; Lembo et al., 1998; McCaul & Malott, 1984; McCaul, Monson, & Maki, 1992; Villemure & Bushnell, 2002). The traditional view might be that distraction simply decreases the patient's awareness of the pain signal; however, distraction may actually attenuate the transmission of nociceptive information resulting in a reduction of pain-related information represented in the brain. For example, attentional modulation was shown to diminish responses of second-order neurons in trigeminal nucleus caudalis as well as in medial thalamus to noxious heat in monkeys (Bushnell, Duncan, Dubner, & He, 1984; Bushnell & Duncan, 1989). More recently, human brain imaging studies revealed that distraction alters pain-related cerebral activation patterns. For example, a vibratory counter stimulus reduced ratings of heat pain and diminished pain-related activation in several brain regions (e.g., anterior cingulate, insula, thalamus) (Longe et al., 2001). Similarly, cognitive distraction reduced heat-pain ratings as well as pain-associated cerebral activation (Bantick et al., 2002). A more recent study demonstrated that distraction attenuated heat-pain ratings and increased activation in the periaqueductal gray (PAG) (Tracey et al., 2002). Interestingly, the degree of pain reduction was correlated with PAG activation, suggesting that the hypoalgesic effects of distraction may be due to activation of opioid-mediated descending analgesic pathways. Thus, distraction is an effective intervention for pain and its neurobiological effects are being elucidated.

drug abuse: *See* ADDICTION.

dysmenorrhea: Dysmenorrhea, or painful menstruation, refers to pelvic pain that can occur immediately before, during, and after menses. Primary dysmenorrhea occurs in the absence of any known disease process or structural abnormality, while secondary dysmenorrhea is associated with some pelvic disease (e.g., endometriosis, pelvic inflammatory disease). Primary dysmenorrhea can be further subdivided into spasmodic versus congestive dysmenorrhea. Spasmodic dysmenorrhea involves acute pain spasms usually restricted to the abdomen, thighs, and lower back, occurring during the first two days of menses. Congestive dysmenorrhea involves more widespread aches and pain (e.g., headache, breast pain, muscle and joint stiffness) as well as nonpain symptoms (e.g., mood disturbance, fatigue), which start before menses and are relieved by onset of menstruation (Dalton, 1969). Dysmenorrhea is extremely common, with prevalence rates well above 50 percent in most studies, and this condition is associated with considerable health care utilization, substantial lost time from work and school, and significant impact on daily activities among sufferers (Banikarim, Chacko, & Kelder, 2000; Hillen, Grbavac, Johnston, Straton, & Keogh, 1999; Zondervan et al., 1998; Harlow & Park, 1996).

Evidence that dysmenorrhea is associated with psychological dysfunction is quite limited (Freeman, Rickels, & Sondheimer, 1993; Bancroft, Williamson, Warner, Rennie, & Smith, 1993). Also, cognitive-behavioral coping skills training produced modest benefit in patients with spadmodic but not congestive dysmenorrhea (Amodei, Nelson, Jarrett, & Sigmon, 1987). Several studies examined pain perception in dysmenorrhea with inconsistent results (Fillingim, 2003). However, the most recent and carefully conducted studies suggest at least some enhancement of pain sensitivity in dysmenorrhea. For example, Giamberardino, Berkley, Iezzi, Debigontina, & Vecchiet (1997) evaluated the influence of menstrual-cycle phase on electrical pain thresholds determined at different body sites (abdomen, arm, leg) and different tissue depths (skin, subcutis, muscle) in dysmenorrheic women. In general, women with dysmenorrhea had lower pain thresholds than controls when tested at subcutis and muscle but not skin, with the greatest group differences emerging when stimuli were applied to the abdominal muscle. More recently, Granot and colleagues (2001) assessed heat-pain perception and pain-evoked potentials in dysmenorrheic women and healthy controls at four menstrual-cycle phases. Heat-pain threshold showed no differences across group or cycle phases; however, dysmenorrheic women rated suprathreshold heat stimuli as more painful compared to controls. Regarding evoked potential, the greatest amplitudes and longest latencies emerged during the follicular phase across both groups, and regardless of cycle phase, women with dysmenorrhea had longer latencies than nondysmenorrheics. The authors interpreted this difference in latency as indicating greater impact of the pain percept on women with dysmenorrhea. Bajaj, Bajaj, Madsen, & Arendt-Nielsen (2002) found that women with dysmenorrhea had lower heat- and pressure-pain thresholds at multiple body sites during the menstrual phase. Thus, enhanced pain sensitivity may be characteristic of dysmenorrhea.

E education: Educational interventions have been investigated for both acute and chronic pain. Regarding patient education, numerous trials examined the effects of preoperative education patients' perioperative outcomes. For example, several studies in patients undergoing joint replacement indicate that presurgical education reduced preoperative anxiety and pain, and may reduce length of hospital stay (Daltroy, Morlino, Eaton, Poss, & Liang, 1998; Giraudet-Le Quintrec et al., 2003; Butler, Hurley, Buchanan, & Smith-VanHorne, 1996; Shuldham, 1999). It is important to recognize that many interventions that are deemed "education" often include other active treatments, especially training in relaxation and other coping skills (e.g., Haugli, Steen, Laerum, Nygard, & Finset, 2001). Therefore, some of the benefits of "education" may actually be due to the use of specific coping strategies.

The effects of educational interventions for chronic pain are somewhat less impressive. In a study of back pain patients, education reduced fear-avoidance beliefs and disability but did not influence pain (Burton, Waddell, Tillotson, & Summerton, 1999). In another trial, education did not reduce disability or improve return to work following a back injury (Hazard, Reid, Haugh, & McFarlane, 2000). Moreover, quantitative and qualitative reviews of education regarding back pain (i.e., Back School) show some short-term benefit in terms of knowledge and improved posture and body mechanics, but minimal effects on pain or health care utilization (Maier-Riehle & Harter, 2001; Koes, van Tulder, van der Windt, & Bouter, 1994). It is also noteworthy that education is an often used active control condition against which other self-management approaches are compared, and although patients in the education condition often show improvements, cognitive-behavioral self-management interventions are typically more effective (Linton & Andersson, 2000; Frost, Klaber Moffett, Moser, & Fairbank, 1995; Ersek, Turner, McCurry, Gibbons, & Kraybill, 2003; Keefe et al., 1996, 1999).

Education for patients experiencing cancer-related pain has shown some benefit. Specifically, educational interventions that include information not only related to pain and pain management but also instruction regarding better communication with health care providers have shown benefit for these patients (de Wit et al., 2001; Oliver, Kravitz, Kaplan, & Meyers, 2001; West et al., 2003). Taken together, these results suggest that education may improve some perioperative outcomes, but education alone is of less benefit than more intensive self-management approaches for chronic pain.

Another component of education is education of providers regarding appropriate pain assessment and treatment. Indeed, educating providers regarding more effective cancer pain management has been effective at improving providers' knowledge and attitudes about pain management, though there may be little impact on patients' pain levels (Allard, Maunsell, Labbe, & Dorval, 2001; Ger et al., 2003). A curriculum in pain management and palliative care was found to improve medical residents' analgesic prescribing patterns (Ury et al., 2002). Similarly, an educational intervention for physicians regarding management of low back pain reduced lost worktime for these patients (Derebery, Giang, Saracino, & Fogarty, 2002). Also, educating physicians and other medical staff regarding reduction in the use of nonsteroidal anti-inflammatory drugs (NSAIDs) in nursing home residents has been effective at decreasing NSAID use (Ray et al., 2001; Stein et al., 2001). These findings indicate that provider education can produce significant improvements in knowledge and attitudes as well as pain-related outcomes.

emotion: As discussed in previous sections, emotional distress is elevated in chronic pain patients compared to controls, and measures of emotional distress are associated with reports of both clinical and experimental pain. Four models explaining the relationship between negative emotion and chronic pain have been proffered (Robinson & Riley, 1999). One explanation is that negative emotion increases pain sensitivity, as previously discussed. Second, negative emotions may cause pain. For example, stress-induced emotions may be accompanied by physiological responses that produce pain (Tsigos & Chrousos, 2002; Flor & Turk, 1989), and some argued that chronic pain may actually be a variant of depression (Blumer & Heilbronn, 1982; Ward et al., 1982). Third, negative emotions occur as a result of chronic pain. Fourth, the association between negative emotion and pain may result from some third variable (e.g., biological changes or severe stress). Each of these possibilities is discussed in more detail in other sections of this book. (*See also* ANGER; ANXIETY; DEPRESSION.)

endogenous opioids: The discovery of endogenous opioid peptides some thirty years ago opened a whole new era of pain research (Hughes, Smith, Kosterlitz, Fothergill, & Morgan, 1975; Terenius, 1975). Indeed the endogenous opioid system represents the most well-characterized pain modulatory system. Endogenous opioids participate substantially in descending pain inhibition (Basbaum & Fields, 1984), and the endogenous opioid system may be influenced by psychological factors. Placebo analgesia, which depends on psychological variables such as expectancy and desire, is one prime example (*see* PLACEBO for complete discussion). In addition, Frid, Singer, & Rana (1979) demonstrated that individuals who perceived an experimental task as challenging and expected to perform well showed a decrease in pain tolerance after administration of naloxone (an opioid antagonist), and those who did not view the pain task as a challenge were unaffected. Also, an experimental study demonstrated that coping-skills training (e.g., relaxation, distraction) increased cold-pressor pain tolerance, and this was partially reversed by naloxone (Bandura, O'Leary, Taylor, Gauthier, & Gossard, 1987). More recently, Bruehl, Burns, Chung, Ward, & Johnson (2002) reported that anger-management style was related to the effects of naloxone on pain perception. Specifically, low scores on anger expression were associated with greater naloxone-induced increases in experimental pain ratings, such that low anger out predicted more robust endogenous opioid influence on pain perception.

ethnicity: Disparities in health across ethnic groups have become a topic of increasing interest in recent years (Byrd & Clayton, 2002), and ethnic differences in the experience of pain has garnered specific attention (Green et al., 2003). Some explanation of terminology is warranted. Most agree that the terms race and ethnicity have different connotations and should not be used interchangeably. Multiple definitions of race have been suggested. Historically, the term race was used to imply biological differences among groups of people who had distinguishing physical characteristics. However, in recent years many experts have eschewed the notion that race is a biological or genetic construct (Bhopal, 1997; Byrd & Clayton, 2002). Thus, race has been defined as, "The group a person belongs to as a result of a mix of physical features, ancestry, and geographical origins, as identified by others, or, increasingly, as self-identified" (Bhopal, 1998, p. 1970). In addition to its debated implication of biological origins, the term race has historical associations with discrimination and prejudice; therefore, the term ethnic group or ethnicity is often preferred in the context of biomedical research (Bhopal & Rankin, 1999). Ethnicity refers to "the group a person belongs to as a result of a mix of cultural factors, including language, diet, religion, ancestry, and race" (Bhopal, 1998, p. 1970).

Increasing clinical evidence suggests that the experience of clinical pain varies across ethnic groups. For example, higher levels of pain have been reported by African Americans and, to a lesser degree, Hispanic Americans compared to non-Hispanic whites with several acute and chronic painful conditions. (For reviews, see Edwards, Fillingim, & Keefe, 2001; Green et al., 2003.) Also, disparities in pain treatment have been identified, such that minority patients are less likely to receive adequate pain medication compared to whites (Edwards et al., 2001; Green et al., 2003). Ethnic differences in laboratory pain responses have also been reported, and the available evidence indicates that African Americans show greater sensitivity to experimentally induced pain than whites (Edwards et al., 2001; Green et al., 2003).

The contribution of psychological factors to ethnic differences in pain response has been suggested by several authors (Edwards et al., 2001; Rollman, 1998; Zatzick & Dimsdale, 1990), though relatively little empirical data exist to address this issue. Bates, Edwards, & Anderson (1993) reported that Hispanic pain patients reported greater pain and a more external locus of control compared to non-Hispanic white patients, and that external locus of control was associated with greater pain. In a study of pain coping among patients with rheumatoid arthritis, no ethnic differences in pain were noted, but African Americans reported greater use of distraction and praying/hoping, while whites reported higher use of ignoring pain and coping statements and a greater perceived ability to control pain (Jordan, Lumley, & Leisen, 1998). In a study of experimental pain perception, African Americans showed higher levels of catastrophizing and hypervigilance, and hypervigilance partially accounted for some of the group differences in pain perception (Campbell, Fillingim, & Edwards, 2005). Psychological factors may also contribute to ethnic group differences in the use of pain treatment. For example, African Americans are less likely to undergo total joint arthroplasty for arthritis, and this difference in mediated in part by African Americans' expectations regarding outcome and their perception that prayer is an effective coping strategy (Ang, Ibrahim, Burant, Siminoff, & Kent, 2002; Ibrahim, Siminoff, Burant, & Kwoh, 2002). Thus, ethnicity is associated with pain responses, and this may be due in part to the contribution of psychological factors.

exaggeration: *See* MALINGERING.

exercise: Physical exercise is an important component of multidisciplinary treatment for chronic pain. Indeed, in one study chronic pain patients demonstrated very poor cardiopulmonary function before treatment and showed substantial increases in indices of physical fitness after a four-week multidisciplinary treatment program (Davis, Fillingim, Doleys, & Davis, 1992). Myriad forms of exercise training have been applied in the management of chronic pain. For low back pain, evidence suggests that exercise provides at least modest clinical benefits (Lahad, Malter, Berg, & Deyo, 1994; van Tulder, Malmivaara, Esmail, & Koes, 2000; Mior, 2001), and exercise is effective in the management of arthritis (Ettinger Jr. et al., 1997; O'Grady, Fletcher, & Ortiz, 2000) and fibromyalgia (Sim & Adams, 2002; Richards & Scott, 2002; Gowans et al., 2001).

Exercise-induced psychological benefits may be equally important for improving clinical outcomes in patients with chronic pain. A robust literature documents benefits such as improved mood, increased cognitive function, and reduced stress reactivity (Seraganian, 1993). In a trial of aerobic exercise, fibromyalgia patients exhibited significant improvements in depression, anxiety, and self-efficacy (Gowans et al., 2001). Similarly, a trial of aerobic exercise did not reduce pain in low back patients, but mood improved significantly as did use of prescription pain medications (Sculco, Paup, Fernhall, & Sculco, 2001). In addition to the mood benefits, exercise may help reduce fear avoidance in patients with chronic pain. (*See* FEAR AVOIDANCE.) Exercise also produces analgesic effects (Droste, Greenlee, Schreck, & Roskamm, 1991; Gurevich, Kohn, & Davis, 1994; Kemppainen, Paalasmaa, Pertovaara, Alila, & Johansson, 1990; Pertovaara, Huopaniemi, Virtanen, & Johansson, 1984), which may confer some clinical pain reduction.

Typically, exercise is only one component of a multidisciplinary approach. Several studies demonstrated that exercise combined with psychological treatments is more effective than exercise alone (Williams, 2003; Nicholas, Wilson, & Goyen, 1992; Busch, Schachter, Peloso, & Bombardier, 2002; Bendix, Bendix, Ostenfeld, Bush, & Andersen, 1995). Thus, exercise is an important component of pain treatment and its benefits are likely partially mediated by psychological effects.

expectancies: Expectancies refer to outcomes or experiences anticipated or predicted by individuals. Expectancies regarding pain are influenced by both organismic and situational factors and expectancies represent important determinants of the pain experience. Expectancies are believed to mediate nocebo and placebo influences on pain (*see* NOCEBO and PLACEBO). Also, people's expectancies regarding the severity of postoperative pain predict actual pain. For example, among women undergoing gynecological surgery preoperative expectations of pain were significantly correlated with postoperative pain reports (Wallace, 1985; Thomas, Robinson, Champion, McKell, & Pell, 1998). Moreover, patients' expectancies regarding their ability to cope with pain predicted ratings of postoperative pain (Bachiocco, Morselli, & Carli, 1993). Similar findings emerged for laboratory-induced pain. In one experiment, subjects' expectations regarding how much pain they would experience and their ability to tolerate pain were correlated with cold-pressor pain tolerance and pain ratings (Lowery, Fillingim, & Wright, 2003). In another study, Sullivan, Rodgers, & Kirsch (2001) found that pain expectancies partially mediated the relationship between catastrophizing and ratings of cold-pressor pain.

Expectancies also influence other clinically important outcomes. For example, in patients undergoing total joint arthroplasty, preoperative expectations regarding pain were a strong predictor of pain and functional status six months after surgery, even after controlling for preoperative pain and education level (Mahomed et al., 2002). Moreover, preoperative expectation of pain and pain relief predicted satisfaction with postoperative pain management (Svensson, Sjostrom, & Haljamae, 2001). One might hypothesize that greater expectations for pain relief would predict more dissatisfaction after surgery; however, this may not be the case. De Groot and colleagues (1999) found that patients who expected no back or leg pain after lumbar surgery reported less disappointment three days postoperatively compared to patients who expected to have pain, even after controlling for pre- and postsurgical pain. Taken together, these findings indicate that expectancies are related to pain-related outcomes; therefore, interventions to alter patients' expectancies may be particularly helpful for managing pain.

experimental pain: *See* PSYCHOPHYSICS.

eye movement desensitization and reprocessing: Eye movement desensitization and reprocessing (EMDR) is a psychological treatment that has primarily been applied to post-traumatic stress disorder (PTSD) and other anxiety disorders. The clinical protocol involves having patients recall traumatic or anxiety-provoking events while focusing their attention on rapid eye movements guided by the therapist. The evidence indicates that EMDR is superior to a no-treatment condition in treating PTSD (Shapiro & Maxfield, 2002); however, the claim that EMDR is superior to other extant treatments for anxiety disorders has been challenged in recent reviews of the literature (Herbert et al., 2000; Lohr, Lilienfeld, Tolin, & Herbert, 1999). EMDR is a rapidly growing therapy, and some authors promoted it as an effective treatment for chronic pain (Grant, 2000; Grant & Threlfo, 2002); however, no controlled studies to support this claim are available. Conclusions regarding the utility of EMDR for chronic pain must await empirical findings.

 factitious disorder: Factitious disorder involves "intentional production or feigning of physical or psychological signs or symptoms" for the purpose of assuming the sick role (American Psychiatric Association, 1994 p. 474). Factitious disorder should be distinguished from malingering, in which external incentives (e.g., economic gain) for the feigning of symptoms are present. Factitious disorder with physical symptoms is also known as Munchausen syndrome. The prevalence of the disorder is not well characterized, though it is considered to be rare (American Psychiatric Association, 1994).

family: Familial factors can be related to pain from several different perspectives. First, several pain disorders show familial aggregation. For example, in a heterogeneous group of chronic pain patients, 59.5 percent reported having a first-degree relative with chronic pain (Katon, Egan, & Miller, 1985). Familial aggregation has been reported for fibromyalgia (FM) (Pellegrino, Waylonis, & Sommer, 1989; Buskila, Neumann, Hazanov, & Carmi, 1996; Buskila & Neumann, 1997), headache (Ottman, Hong, & Lipton, 1993; Messinger, Spierings, Vincent, & Lebbink, 1991; Ehde, Holm, & Metzger, 1991; Turkat, Kuczmierczyk, & Adams, 1984). Several findings suggest that a family history of pain is associated with increased risk for pain in community-based samples (Edwards, Zeichner, Kuczmierczyk, & Boczkowski, 1985; Koutantji, Pearce, & Oakley, 1998; Lester, Lefebvre, & Keefe, 1994; Sternbach, 1986). Interestingly, a family history of pain has been associated with increased pain sensitivity, especially among women (Fillingim, Edwards, & Powell, 2000; Neumann & Buskila, 1997). These familial influences on risk for clinical pain and sensitivity to experimental pain could be due to genetic influences, social learning, or (more likely) both. The influence of genetics and social learning are discussed in separate sections.

Second, chronic pain can have significant influence on family functioning. Specifically, numerous studies reported increased psychological distress among spouses or partners of individuals with chronic pain, and relationship adjustment is often lower among dyads in which one partner has chronic pain, though this is not always the case (Romano & Schmaling, 2001). Also, chronic pain in children has been shown to adversely affect familial quality of life (Palermo, 2000; Merlijn et al., 2003; Hunfeld et al., 2001, 2002), and chronic pain can negatively impact patients' perceived ability to fulfill family roles (Barlow, Cullen, Foster, Harrison, & Wade, 1999). A number of studies assessed family environment and cohesion in families of patients with chronic pain. Romano and Schmaling (2001) reviewed these findings and concluded that the family environments of individuals with chronic pain tend to be less cohesive, more conflictual, and engaged less in active recreation together compared to healthy families.

Third, familial factors are important predictors of patients' pain-related adjustment. One factor that has been heavily investigated is spousal solicitousness, which refers to the tendency of a patient's spouse to respond to his or her pain behavior with excessive attention and reinforcement. In one study, spousal presence was associated with greater pain reports only for patients who described their spouses as solicitous (Block, Kremer, & Gaylor, 1980). Relatedly, Gil, Keefe, Crisson, & Van Dalfsen (1987) found that higher patient ratings of satisfaction with social support were associated with higher levels of overt pain behavior. Similar associations between spousal solicitousness and increased pain, disability, and pain behavior have been reported by other investigators (Flor, Kerns, & Turk, 1987; Lousberg, Schmidt, & Groenman, 1992; Williamson, Robinson, & Melamed, 1997). Interestingly, spousal solicitousness may influence pain sensitivity in patients. Flor, Breitenstein, Birbaumer, & Furst (1995) found that chronic pain patients who rated their spouses as high in solicitousness showed lower cold-pressor pain tolerance when the spouse was present versus absent, while spouse presence had no impact on pain tolerance in patients with low solicitous spouses. These investigators recently demonstrated that the presence of a solicitous spouse was associated with enhanced brain responses to electrical pain stimulation among low back pain patients, but no such association was found in patients whose spouses were not solicitous (Flor, Lutzenberger, Knost, Diesch, & Birbaumer, 2002). Marital satisfaction and negative spousal responses to pain have been associated with greater symptoms of anxiety and depression among chronic pain patients (Romano & Schmaling, 2001).

One factor that may influence the relationship of familial factors to chronic pain is gender. A stronger relationship has been reported between patient and spouse dysfunction when patients are male (and spouses female) than when patients are female (and spouses male) (Romano, Turner, & Clancy, 1989), suggesting that wives of male patients are more affected by their husbands' pain and dysfunction than are husbands of female patients. In addition, marital dissatisfaction was associated with greater pain, disability, and psychological distress in female but not male chronic pain patients (Saarijarvi, Rytokoski, & Karppi, 1990). Relatedly, punishing spousal responses were associated with increased pain and interference among male patients, but this association was not present for female patients (Burns, Johnson, Mahoney, Devine, & Pawl, 1996). In contrast, spousal criticism contributed to increased affective distress in both women and men with rheumatoid arthritis (Kraaimaat, Van Dam-Baggen, & Bijlsma, 1995). Spousal solicitousness is associated with pain severity and self-reported disability for male patients, is related to lower pain tolerance, poorer functional performance, and increased likelihood of opioid use in females (Fillingim, Doleys, Edwards, & Lowery, 2003).

Multidisciplinary treatment of chronic pain often incorporates family involvement; however, few controlled studies investigated the effectiveness of family therapy for patients with chronic pain. Keefe and colleagues (1996) compared the effectiveness of spouse assisted cognitive behavioral coping skills training (SA-CST) to CST alone and an arthritis education-spousal support (AE-SS) control condition for patients with knee osteoarthritis. They reported that patients in the SA-CST condition showed significantly greater decreases in pain, pain behavior, and psychological distress and increases in pain coping, self-efficacy, and marital adjustment compared to the control condition. Patients in the CST alone group showed similar but somewhat less robust improvements on most measures. A similar pattern of results was observed at the 12-month follow-up (Keefe et al., 1999).

In summary, familial factors are important to consider when evaluating and treating patients with chronic pain. The presence of pain can substantially impact family functioning, and familial responses are predictive of patients' pain-related adjustment. Additional research to determine the effectiveness of family therapy in the treatment of chronic pain is needed.

fatigue: Fatigue refers to decreased energy and a feeling of tiredness. The symptom of fatigue is highly comorbid with pain and has received increased attention. A recent structured review concluded strongly that an association exists between chronic pain and fatigue and that the evidence supports an etiological relationship, such that pain causes fatigue (Fishbain et al., 2003). The studies reviewed included chronic pain from multiple conditions, including fibromyalgia, cancer, headache, arthritis, low back pain, mixed chronic pain, and community samples. Therefore, the association appears not to be restricted to specific diagnoses. Multiple mechanisms could explain the association of fatigue and chronic pain, including sleep disturbance, physical deconditioning, neuroendocrine dysfunction, medication effects, and psychological influences. These findings demonstrate the need to address fatigue as a potentially important treatment target among patients with chronic pain.

fear avoidance: Fear avoidance refers to "the avoidance of movements or activities based on fear" and is believed to contribute significantly to the development of long-term disability associated with musculoskeletal pain (Vlaeyen & Linton, 2000, p. 317). One model of fear avoidance is based on a combination of classical and operant conditioning (*see* BEHAVIORAL FACTORS) (Vlaeyen & Linton, 2000). Specifically, shortly after an injury, physical activity (e.g., bending and lifting) may directly produce pain which then elicits sympathetic activation along with fear, anxiety, and muscle tension. Subsequently, physical activity has become classically conditioned so that it now elicits the fear response independent of pain, which causes the individual to avoid activity. This avoidance of activity reduces fear and anxiety, which provides reinforcement for the avoidant behavior. Vlaeyen incorporated cognitive factors into this behavioral model, such that the fear of injury or pain is accompanied by negative thinking (e.g., catastrophizing), heightened awareness of somatic cues (i.e., hypervigilance), and excessive appraisal of physical activities as dangerous (Vlaeyen & Linton, 2000). Of course, activity avoidance can lead to physical deconditioning, which can increase the likelihood that future activity will be unpleasant and difficult.

Several instruments are available for assessment of pain-related fear, and the most commonly used are: the Fear-Avoidance Beliefs Questionnaire (Waddell, Newton, Henderson, Somerville, & Main, 1993); the Pain Anxiety Symptoms Scale (McCracken, Zayfert, & Gross, 1992); and the Tampa Scale for Kinesiophobia (Kori, 1990). Patients with a high level of pain-related fear also report heightened awareness of somatic symptoms (Vlaeyen & Linton, 2000). Moreover, numerous studies demonstrated that pain-related fear is associated with poorer performance on physical tasks and with greater self-reported pain-related disability (Vlaeyen & Linton, 2000), and fear-avoidance beliefs have been associated with decreased likelihood of return to work after acute back injury (Fritz & George, 2002; Fritz, George, & Delitto, 2001).

Interventions to reduce fear avoidance have been developed and evaluated. In vivo exposure is the cornerstone of treatments to reduce fear avoidance. That is, patients must engage in feared activities. Graded exposure intervention includes educating the patient regarding the fear-avoidance model and the patient develops a hierarchy of fear-eliciting activities, which he or she then practices. In a series of single-case studies, Vlaeyen and colleagues provided evidence supporting the effectiveness of graded exposure to activity in reducing pain-related fear in patients with chronic low back pain (Vlaeyen, de Jong, Geilen, Heuts, & van Breukelen, 2001; Vlaeyen, de Jong, Geilen, Heuts, & van Breukelen, 2002). Specifically, greater reductions in pain-related fear, catastrophizing, and disability emerge with graded exposure compared to only graded activity. A recent clinical trial with acute low back pain found that the effects of graded exposure are moderated by patients' level of fear-avoidance beliefs (George, Fritz, Bialosky, & Donald, 2003). Specifically, graded-exposure based physical therapy produced greater reductions in disability than standard therapy for patients high in fear avoidance; however, patients with low fear avoidance did not benefit from the graded exposure intervention. Thus, treatment to directly address fear avoidance has shown significant clinical efficacy, especially among patients with high levels of pain-related fear.

fibromyalgia: Fibromyalgia (FM) is a rheumatologic disorder of unknown pathophysiology characterized by widespread pain and tenderness to manual palpation. FM had a reported prevalence of 2 percent in one study and 3.3 percent in another, and the female to male ratio is at least 3 to 1 in the general population (White, Speechley, Harth, & Ostbye, 1999; Wolfe, Ross, Anderson, Russell, & Hebert, 1995). In addition to widespread pain, features of FM include fatigue, sleep disturbance, and psychological distress. FM patients exhibit a generalized enhancement of sensitivity to experimentally induced pain. For example, lower thresholds for mechanical pain at both tender and control points have been reported in FM patients compared to controls (Lautenbacher, Rollman, & McCain, 1994; Mountz et al., 1995), and hyperalgesia to other noxious stimuli, including heat and electrical pain, has also been observed (Hurtig, Raak, Kendall, Gerdle, & Wahren, 2001; Kosek, Ekholm, & Hansson, 1996; Lautenbacher et al., 1994). The mechanisms underlying this generalized hypersensitivity have not been elucidated, central alterations in nociceptive processing have been implicated (Staud, 2002). Heightened levels of substance P in the cerebrospinal fluid of FM patients were reported (Bradley et al., 1996; Russell et al., 1994). Also, impairment of endogenous pain inhibition has been documented in FM patients (Kosek & Hansson, 1997; Lautenbacher & Rollman, 1997). Recent findings indicate enhanced temporal summation of pain in patients with FM, further implicating central nervous system involvement (Staud, Vierck, Cannon, Mauderli, & Price, 2001). In addition, FM patients show altered cerebral blood flow in brain regions involved in nociceptive processing both at rest (Mountz et al., 1995) and during painful stimulation (Gracely, Petzke, Wolf, & Clauw, 2002). Staud and colleagues (2003) also reported that painful aftersensations following repetitive heat stimuli significantly predicted patients' self-reported clinical pain, suggesting that this experimental measure of hypersensitivity is clinically relevant. Several lines of evidence suggest abnormal central nervous system processing of noxious stimuli among individuals with FM.

Psychological factors have been widely investigated in FM. Fibromyalgia has been associated with elevated levels of psychological distress (Gur et al., 2002; White, Nielson, Harth, Ostbye, & Speechley, 2002; Walker et al., 1997); hypervigilance (McDermid, Rollman, & McCain, 1996); and catastrophizing (Geisser et al., 2003). Bradley and colleagues (1996) compared FM patients recruited from clinical settings to community-based individuals who met diagnostic criteria for FM but had not sought treatment for their symptoms (i.e., FM nonpatients). FM patients reported higher levels of psychological distress and greater pain compared to nonpatients (Kersh et al., 2001), and the frequency of psychiatric disorders was greater in FM patients versus nonpatients, and the latter did not differ from pain-free controls (Aaron et al., 1996). Also, physical or emotional trauma preceding the onset of FM symptoms and/or treatment was associated with more health care seeking and greater disability but not with pain severity or pain threshold (Aaron et al., 1997). These findings suggest that psychological factors may not be etiologic but may contribute to health care seeking in FM.

A number of controlled and uncontrolled trials examined the utility of psychological treatment for FM. Early uncontrolled studies showed promising results (White & Nielson, 1995; Nielson, Walker, & McCain, 1992); however, these effects must be interpreted cautiously as several studies suggest that a substantial proportion of FM patients show symptomatic improvements over time with standard care (Granges, Zilko, & Littlejohn, 1994; Fitzcharles, Costa, & Poyhia, 2003). Meta-analytic reviews suggest that psychological treatments may provide modest improvement in FM symptoms, though relatively few controlled trials of psychological interventions for FM are available (Rossy et al., 1999; Sim & Adams, 2002). Some argue that combining cognitive-behavioral treatment with exercise may enhance the effectiveness of both (Williams, 2003). Important directions for future research include determining optimal treatment combinations and identifying patient characteristics that should be used to tailor treatment regimens.

functional assessment: Functional impairment represents a major concern among patients with chronic pain, and assessment of functional status is an important aspect of patient evaluation. Multiple methods are available to quantify function among patients with chronic pain, including assessment of: range of motion, trunk strength, lifting capacity, aerobic fitness, and numerous task-specific tests (Polatin & Mayer, 2001). One application of quantitative functional assessment is detecting a submaximal or insincere effort as an index of malingering. However, two recent reviews found little evidence that submaximal efforts are more variable than maximal efforts, and numerous factors (other than malingering) can influence performance on functional tests (Fishbain, Cutler, Rosomoff, & Rosomoff, 1999; Robinson & Dannecker, 2003). For example, several studies demonstrated significant correlations between psychological variables (e.g., fear avoidance, self-efficacy, pain coping, depression) and functional performance (Ruan, Haig, Geisser, Yamakawa, & Buchholz, 2001; Al Obaidi, Nelson, Al Awadhi, & Al Shuwaie, 2000; Lackner & Carosella, 1999). Thus, there appears to be little evidence that functional testing can be used to detect malingering, but psychological factors are important predictors of function. However, assessment of functional status is an important outcome measure for detecting clinically important effects of treatments. Given that performance-based functional tests and self-report instruments of disability have only modest overlap, performance on functional tasks remains an important measure of clinical status in patients with chronic pain (Lee, Simmonds, Novy, & Jones, 2001; Reneman, Jorritsma, Schellekens, & Goeken, 2002; Simmonds et al., 1998).

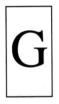

gate control theory: The paper by Melzack and Wall (Melzack & Wall, 1965) in which they presented the gate control theory of pain was perhaps the single most important publication in the modern history of pain research. In their seminal paper, Melzack and Wall review clinical, psychological, and physiological evidence that refutes the tenets of specificity theory, which proposed a highly specialized system in which specific "pain receptors" transmitted pain signals to a pain center in the brain. They then reviewed pattern theory, which, in contrast to specificity theory, proposed that sensory receptors were entirely nonspecific and that the experience of pain was created by central summation of sensory information due to stimulus intensity. Melzack and Wall also lucidly presented the shortcomings of pattern theory. The gate control theory incorporated both the physiological specialization of specificity theory and the central summation of pattern theory.

In short, the gate control theory proposed that (1) the substantia gelatinosa in the dorsal horn modulates afferent patterns before they act upon transmission (T) cells; (2) the pattern of afferent activity in the dorsal column system activates brain processes that influence the gate control system via descending control and (3) the T cells activate neural mechanisms that lead to pain perception and responses. One example of pain modulation was the inhibitory influence of large fiber (i.e., A-beta mechanocreceptor) input, which gave way to the development of therapies such as transcutaneous electrical nerve stimulation. However, from a psychological perspective, the importance of the gate control theory was its assertion that psychological factors produce descending influences on the gate control system. Indeed, Melzack and Wall (1965) state, "The model suggests that psychological factors such as past experience, attention, and emotion influence pain response and perception by acting on the gate control system" (p. 978). Thus, the gate control theory for the first time legitimized the neurobiology of psychological influences on pain, and the ensuing four decades supported the assertion that psychological factors do indeed alter pain transmission.

gender: The issue of gender differences in pain has received dramatically increasing attention in recent years (Fillingim, 2000). Considerable evidence suggests that women experience more frequent clinical pain than men. For example, women are at increased risk for developing several chronic painful disorders, including temporomandibular disorders, fibromyalgia, migraine headache, irritable bowel syndrome, and joint pain, and population surveys reveal more frequent pain among women than men in the community (Fillingim, 2003; LeResche, 1999; Unruh, 1996). Laboratory-based studies indicate that women exhibit greater sensitivity to experimentally induced pain than men across a variety of stimulus modalities and assessment methods (Berkley, 1997; Fillingim & Maixner, 1995; Riley, Robinson, Wise, Myers, & Fillingim, 1998). Some of these findings are based on subjective responses, such that women have lower pain thresholds and tolerances and generally describe noxious stimuli as more painful. However, gender differences are reported in more sophisticated measures as well. For example, women display greater temporal summation of thermal and mechanical pain, which is thought to depend on sensitization of central neurons subserving pain transmission (Fillingim, Maixner, Kincaid, & Silva, 1998; Sarlani & Greenspan, 2002). Further, the nociceptive flexion reflex, which is a spinal pain-related muscle response, occurs in women at a lower stimulus intensity than in men (France & Suchowiecki, 1999), and women showed greater pupil dilation in response to mechanical pain than men (Ellermeier & Westphal, 1995). Recent studies used functional brain imaging to examine pain-related cerebral activation across sexes. The findings reveal some gender differences in brain responses to pain; however, the pattern of results differs across studies, with women showing greater pain-related activation in some brain regions, men showing greater activation in other regions, and no sex differences in some areas (Derbyshire, Nichols, Firestone, Townsend, & Jones, 2002; Naliboff et al., 2003; Paulson, Minoshima, Morrow, & Casey, 1998). These sex differences in clinical and experimental pain responses are inevitably determined by interactions among multiple biopsychosocial variables, including psychological and social factors (e.g., mood, pain coping, sex roles) as well as biological variables (e.g., sex steroids, genetics).

Sex differences in treatment responses have also been reported. Regarding pharmacologic responses, numerous findings suggest that there may be sex differences in responses to analgesic medications (Craft, 2003; Fillingim & Gear, 2004). The results, in general, suggest that women display more robust analgesic responses to opioids, and too few studies with nonopioid analgesics are available to draw firm conclusions. Sex differences in response to nonpharmacologic interventions for pain have received less empirical attention. In the laboratory setting, a cognitive intervention that instructed subjects to focus on the pain sensations they experienced was effective for reducing pain intensity in men but not women (Keogh, Hatton, & Ellery, 2000). Also, women but not men reported lower ratings of cold-pressor pain after exercising on a treadmill, while men but not women showed reduced pain ratings after playing video games (Sternberg, Bokat, Kass, Alboyadjian, & Gracely, 2001). In the clinical setting, conventional physical therapy was more effective for men, while intensive dynamic back exercises produced better pain reduction among women (Hansen et al., 1993). Women showed greater improvements following multidisciplinary treatment for facial and back pain (Krogstad, Jokstad, Dahl, & Vassend, 1996; Jensen, Bergstrom, Ljungquist, Bodin, & Nygren, 2001). Other clinical studies reported similar treatment responses gains for women and men following active rehabilitation for chronic low back pain (Kankaanpaa, Taimela, Airaksinen, & Hanninen, 1999; Mannion et al., 2001).

In addition to these quantitative sex differences, accumulating evidence points to potentially important differences in the mediators of pain responses among women and men. For example, in healthy young adults, higher self-efficacy was associated with lower experimental pain sensitivity in females but not males, while higher anxiety predicted greater pain sensitivity only in males (Fillingim, Keefe, Light, Booker, & Maixner, 1996). These findings were subsequently supported in clinical populations, such that pain-related anxiety was associated with increased pain and self-reported disability in men but not women with chronic pain (Edwards, Augustson, & Fillingim, 2000), and lower self-efficacy for controlling and decreasing pain was associated with greater disability among women but not men with chronic low back pain (Mannion et al., 2001). Mediators of treatment outcome may also differ across genders. Burns, Johnson, Devine, Mahoney, & Pawl (1998) reported that measures of anger expression and suppression predicted with treatment responses among males but not females. Similarly, pain-relatred anxiety predicted greater improvements from interventional and cognitive-behavioral treatment among males but not females (Edwards, Augustson, & Fillingim, 2003). These results illustrate the wide range of sex differences in pain-related responses and suggest that the gender of the patient may be an important determinant of pain perception and treatment outcome.

genetics: Advances in understanding the human genome have led to an explosion of biomedical research on the genetics of disease and complex human traits, including pain. Indeed, some proportion of the substantial interindividual differences that characterize clinical and experimental pain responses is due to genetic factors. Pain genetics lags behind many of fields of genetics in biomedicine. However, many pain conditions show familial aggregation, including fibromyalgia (Pellegrino, Waylonis, & Sommer, 1989; Buskila, Neumann, Hazanov, & Carmi, 1996; Buskila & Neumann, 1997); headache (Ottman, Hong, & Lipton, 1993; Messinger, Spierings, Vincent, & Lebbink, 1991; Ehde, Holm, & Metzger, 1991; Turkat, Kuczmierczyk, & Adams, 1984; Aromaa, Sillanpaa, Rautava, & Helenius, 2000); irritable bowel syndrome (Kalantar, Locke, Zinsmeister, Beighley, & Talley, 2003; Kalantar et al., 2003; Levy et al., 2001) and a heterogeneous sample of chronic pain sufferers (Katon, Egan, & Miller, 1985). Self-reported family history of pain is also associated with frequency of pain complaints in population-based samples (Edwards, Zeichner, Kuczmierczyk, & Boczkowski, 1985; Koutantji, Pearce, & Oakley, 1998; Lester, Lefebvre, & Keefe, 1994; Sternbach, 1986). Of course, these familial associations could be explained by environmental or genetic factors (or more likely an interaction between the two).

Laboratory research in experimental animals reveals significant heritability for measure of basal nociceptive response as well and responses to analgesic agents (Mogil, 1999). Human studies of genetic influences on pain perception are less abundant. Pressure-pain threshold was determined in monozygotic and dizygotic twins and showed a heritability of only 10 percent (Macgregor, Griffiths, Baker, & Spector, 1997). Recently, investigators explored associations between pain sensitivity and single nucleotide polymorphisms (SNP) of specific genes. One such experiment revealed heritability estimates of 22 to 46 percent across three pain modalities and found an association of a δ-opioid receptor gene *(OPRD1)* SNP with thermal pain responses among men but not women (Kim et al., 2003), consistent with the results of a previous linkage mapping study in mice (Mogil et al., 1997). Zubieta and colleagues (2003) reported that a SNP of the catechol-*O*-methyltransferase gene *(COMT)* was associated with both pain report and pain-induced brain μ-opioid receptor binding using an experimental muscle pain induction. Thus, some limited evidence exists of genetic contributions to human pain responses.

Interestingly, most major aspects of psychological functioning (e.g., personality, cognitive abilities, affect) show substantial heritability (Exton, Artz, Siffert, & Schedlowski, 2003; Eid, Riemann, Angleitner, & Borkenau, 2003; Bouchard Jr. & McGue, 2003); therefore, genetic factors could influence pain responses indirectly through their effects on psychological processes. Indeed, it has recently been reported that fibromyalgia patients were more likely to be homozygous for the rare allele of a SNP in the promoter region of the serotonin transporter gene, and FM patients showing this genotype showed greater psychological distress than patients with other genotypes (Offenbaecher et al., 1999). Thus, a genotype associated with a pain disorder is also related to psychological functioning. Undoubtedly future research will help elucidate the role of genetics in the experience of pain.

group therapy: Group therapy is a frequently used treatment modality for patients with chronic pain. Yalom (1985) identified multiple therapeutic factors that characterize group therapy, and many of these are operational in cognitive-behavioral group therapy for chronic pain, including: instillation of hope, universality (i.e., patients realize that others have similar problems), imparting information, altruism (i.e., patients benefit from helping each other), development of social skills, imitative behavior (i.e., observational learning). Keefe and colleagues (1996) describe several types of group treatments for pain, including education groups, support groups, and behavior-change groups. These authors also provide an excellent description of a cognitive behavioral group treatment program designed to impart pain coping skills. Group therapy is an optimal modality for delivering psychological interventions to patients with chronic pain.

headache: Headache represents the most common pain complaint in the primary care setting and is among the most common presenting symptoms in the emergency department (Hasse, Ritchey, & Smith, 2002; McCaig & Burt, 2003). The two most common headache diagnoses are migraine and tension-type headache. Diagnostic criteria for migraine include: headaches lasting 4 to 72 hours; two or more of the following—unilateral, pulsating, moderate to severe intensity, aggravated by physical activity; and nausea/vomiting or photophobia/phonophobia occur during headache. Migraine can occur with or without aura, which refers to prodromal symptoms, including visual symptoms, sensory symptoms, or speech disturbance (Headache Classification Committee of the International Headache Society, 1988; Headache Classification Committee of the International Headache Society, 2004). Migraine prevalence is approximately 18 percent in females and 6 percent in males (Lipton et al., 2002; Lipton, Stewart, Diamond, Diamond, & Reed, 2001). Tension-type headache (TTH) refers to headaches lasting from 30 minutes to seven days, which are described as pressing/tightening, mild to moderate in intensity, bilateral, and unaffected by physical activity. Also, nausea and vomiting are not associated. TTH can be episodic (i.e., <15 headaches per month) or chronic (>15 per month) (Headache Classification Committee of the International Headache Society, 1988; Headache Classification Committee of the International Headache Society, 2004). Episodic TTH is quite common, with lifetime prevalence ranging from 30 to78 percent (Jensen, 2003; Ho & Ong, 2003). One-year prevalence of episodic TTH was reported to be 38 percent and slightly higher among women than men (Schwartz, Stewart, Simon, & Lipton, 1998). Chronic TTH occurs in 2 to 3 percent of the population, more commonly in women than men (Jensen, 2003; Ho & Ong, 2003).

Historically, headache sufferers were described as having specific personality traits, though minimal evidence supports the concept of a headache-prone personality (Holroyd & Lipchik, 1999; Silberstein, Lipton, & Breslau, 1995). However, comorbidity between migraine and psychopathology, especially depression and anxiety disorders, has been reported (Breslau, Lipton, Stewart, Schultz, & Welch, 2003; Breslau et al., 2000; Breslau, Schultz, Stewart, Lipton, & Welch, 2001; Puca et al., 1999; Silberstein, Lipton, & Breslau, 1995). As mentioned earlier (*see* DEPRESSION), Breslau and colleagues (2000, 2003) reported a bidirectional relationship between major depression and migraine headache, such that each increases risk for the other. However, the relationship of nonmigraine severe headache to major depression was unidirectional, with headache increasing risk of depression but not the reverse (Breslau et al., 2000). Stress is commonly reported by headache patients and represents a significant precipitant of migraine and tension headache episodes (Puca et al., 1999; Fernandez & Sheffield, 1996; Rasmussen, 1993). Another common aggravating factor in headaches is medication overuse, also known as rebound headache (Diener & Katsarava, 2001; Fritsche & Diener, 2002; Limmroth, Katsarava, Fritsche, Przywara, & Diener, 2002).

Psychological treatments for headache disorders have been widely investigated. Both systematic and qualitative reviews of clinical trials of behavioral therapy for headache disorders support its efficacy, and in general these treatments produce a 40 to 60 percent reduction in headache activity for both migraine and TTH (Eccleston, Yorke, Morley, Williams, & Mastroyannopoulou, 2003; Haddock et al., 1997; Holroyd & Penzien, 1990b; Lipchik, Holroyd, & Nash, 2002). Important components of cognitive-behavioral treatment for headache include relaxation, identifying headache precipitants, education regarding medication use, cognitive restructuring for stress control, use of specific coping techniques (e.g., distraction, imagery, reinterpretation of pain), and possibly thermal biofeedback (Lipchik et al., 2002).

hyperalgesia: Hyperalgesia refers to an increased pain response to a previously painful stimulus (Merskey & Bogduk, 1994). Hyperalgesia is characteristic of several clinical pain states, including inflammatory pain, neuropathic pain, and complex regional pain syndrome. As with allodynia, hyperalgesia can be produced by peripheral and/or central sensitization processes. In clinical settings, hyperalgesia has often been mistaken for overly dramatic or exaggerated pain responding by the patient, when a neurobiological explanation is present for the enhanced pain sensitivity.

hypertension: The relevance of hypertension to pain may not be obvious to many readers; however, substantial literature demonstrates that hypertension is associated with decreased pain sensitivity. The first studies to document this phenomenon observed increased latencies to display nociceptive responses in experimentally and spontaneously hypertensive rats (Maixner, Touw, Brody, Gebhart, & Long, 1982; Zamir & Segal, 1979; Zamir, Segal, & Simantov, 1980). These findings were initially replicated in humans by Zamir & Shuber (1980), and numerous subsequent studies have reported that hypertensive humans show diminished pain sensitivity compared to normotensives (France, 1999; Ghione, 1996). In fact, even among normotensives, higher resting blood pressure is associated with lower pain sensitivity (Bruehl, Carlson, & McCubbin, 1992; Fillingim & Maixner, 1996; France, 1999). Blood pressure and other cardiovascular responses represent mechanisms for ongoing pain inhibition, and there is evidence that these inhibitory systems are dysregulated in some patients with chronic pain (Bruehl, McCubbin, & Harden, 1999; Maixner, Fillingim, Kincaid, Sigurdsson, & Harris, 1997). Also, psychological factors may alter the relationship between cardiovascular responses and pain perception. For example, experimental manipulations of incentive and perceived ability influenced the relationship between blood pressure responses and pain perception (Fillingim, Browning, Powell, & Wright, 2002; Lowery, Fillingim, & Wright, 2003).

hypervigilance: Hypervigilance refers to increased awareness of and reactivity to aversive or unpleasant sensory stimuli. Related terms include somatization and perceptual amplification. Chapman (1978) first introduced the term hypervigilance into the pain literature, which he defined as a constant scanning of the body for somatic and, particularly, pain sensations. Hypervigilance has been operationalized in several ways. For example, it can be assessed using psychometric instruments, such as the Pain Vigilance and Awareness Questionnaire (McCracken, 1997) or the Pennebaker Inventory of Limbic Languidness (Pennebaker, 1982). Alternatively, laboratory measures of attentional control have been used to measure hypervigilance. Specifically, the influence of pain (or other noxious sensory stimuli) on an individuals' performance on a concurrent attention demanding cognitive task is believed to reflect heightened attention (i.e., hypervigilance) to the painful sensation. Questionnaire studies revealed elevated scores on measures of hypervigilance in fibromyalgia patients and patients with rheumatoid arthritis relative to pain-free controls (McDermid, Rollman, & McCain, 1996). Also, self-report measures of somatization predict the development of chronic widespread pain (McBeth, Macfarlane, Benjamin, & Silman, 2001; McBeth, Macfarlane, Hunt, & Silman, 2001). In an experiment combining both questionnaire and laboratory assessment approaches, Eccleston, Crombez, Aldrich, & Stannard (1997) measured somatic awareness in 46 chronic pain patients and then had them perform an attentionally demanding reaction time task. The results indicated that pain intensity and somatic awareness interacted to affect task performance, such that patients with high pain levels and high somatic awareness had the poorest performance. Hypervigilance is also associated with higher levels of pain-related fear and catastrophizing (Roelofs, Peters, McCracken, & Vlaeyen, 2003). Although hypervigilance is typically conceptualized at the psychological/behavioral level, it seems likely that neurobiological changes underlie hypervigilance, though they have yet to be fully elucidated.

hypnosis: Hypnosis has been used in biomedicine for centuries, but modern hypnosis dates back most notably to the work of Dr. Franz Anton Mesmer in the late 1700s (Barber, 1996). Among hypnotic phenomena, hypnotic analgesia is perhaps the most impressive and has the greatest empirical support. Hypnosis has been defined as "an altered condition or state of consciousness characterized by a markedly increased receptivity to suggestion, the capacity for modification of perception and memory, and the potential for systematic control of a variety of physiological functions" (Barber, 1996, p. 5).

Hypnosis classically includes an induction phase, which often includes relaxation, followed by suggestions. Despite its somewhat mystical connotations, substantial evidence supports the use of hypnosis in the treatment of pain.

Several quantitative and qualitative review articles report that hypnosis is an effective method for pain reduction in a variety of clinical settings, including experimental pain, acute clinical pain, and chronic pain (Astin, 2004; Holden, Deichmann, & Levy, 1999; Montgomery, DuHamel, & Redd, 2000; Pan, Morrison, Ness, Fugh-Berman, & Leipzig, 2000; Patterson & Jensen, 2003; Sellick & Zaza, 1998). Patterson and Jensen (2003) discuss several important methodological issues to consider when interpreting the clinical effects of hypnosis. First, individuals high in hypnotic suggestibility may benefit more from hypnosis, but hypnotic suggestibility can improve with training. Second, it is important to distinguish the specific from the nonspecific effects of hypnosis, including the specific suggestions provided by the therapist as well as ensuring that the control condition is well-matched to the hypnotic condition for therapist time and patient expectancies. Third, the dose effects of hypnosis are not well understood. For example, do longer hypnotic sessions and more frequent home practice confer greater clinical effects? Moreover, are there cumulative dose effects, such that the benefits increase over time with practice?

Although evidence suggests that hypnosis is superior to control conditions in reducing pain, whether hypnosis is more effective than other psychological interventions (e.g., relaxation) for pain control is less clear. Patterson and Jensen (2003) conclude that hypnosis is superior to other psychological treatments in reducing acute pain but not for chronic pain, though this latter finding may be due to the simplistic approach that many studies have taken in applying hypnosis to chronic pain. Regarding acute pain, hypnosis was compared to stress management in 60 patients undergoing plastic surgery; the stress management condition included relaxation training, emotional support, and cognitive coping skills (Faymonville et al., 1997). Compared to the stress-management group, the hypnosis group reported lower anxiety, less intraoperative and postoperative pain, required less sedation (midazolam, alfentanil), and showed less intraoperative physiological activation. Regarding experimentally induced pain, in addition to its effects on reported pain, hypnosis has been found to reduce pain-related muscle reflexes and to alter cerebral responses to pain (Faymonville et al., 2000; Kiernan, Dane, Phillips, & Price, 1995; Rainville et al., 1999; Rainville, Duncan, Price, Carrier, & Bushnell, 1997).

Thus, it seems evident that hypnosis is among the most effective psychological modalities for the treatment of many types of pain. However, there remains considerable disagreement regarding the mechanisms whereby hypnosis exerts its clinical effects.

hypochondriasis: Hypochondriasis technically refers to a psychiatric disorder in which the patient has a preoccupation with the idea or fear that she or he has a serious disease based on misinterpretation of bodily symptoms (American Psychiatric Association, 1994). Hypochondriasis is characterized by excessive preoccupation with physical symptoms and somatic functioning. Although the disorder is relatively rare in the general population, hypochrondriacal features (i.e., excessive concern or worry regarding somatic symptoms) are fairly prevalent and are likely to be overrepresented in chronic pain populations (Rief, Hessel, & Braehler, 2001).

hysteria: *See* CONVERSION DISORDER.

I

Irritable bowel syndrome: Irritable bowel syndrome (IBS) is a gastrointestinal disorder characterized by abdominal pain or discomfort associated with altered bowel habits (Thompson et al., 1999). IBS is classified as constipation-predominant or diarrhea-predominant based on the nature of the bowel disturbance. The prevalence of IBS is approximately 15 percent in Western populations, and women are more commonly affected, with IBS occurring approximately twice as often among women than men (Drossman, Whitehead, & Camilleri, 1997; Talley, 1999). Despite the fact that only a minority of individuals with the disorder seek treatment, IBS is one of the most common gastrointestinal disorders seen by physicians in the primary care setting, and is responsible for up to 40 percent of referrals to gastroenterologists (Drossman et al., 1997; Talley, 1999).

One hallmark of IBS is visceral hypersensitivity, such that IBS patients display a decreased pain threshold in response to rectal or colonic distention (Mertz, Naliboff, Munakata, Niazi, & Mayer, 1995).

IBS patients often report multiple extraintestinal complaints, including headache, musculoskeletal pain, fatigue, and psychological symptoms (Mayer & Gebhart, 1994; Whitehead, Palsson, & Jones, 2002). Given these generalized somatic complaints, whether IBS patients also demonstrate enhanced sensitivity to somatic stimuli has been investigated. Some findings suggest that IBS patients are no more sensitive to experimentally induced somatic pain than healthy controls (Chang, Mayer, Johnson, FitzGerald, & Naliboff, 2000), while others have reported enhanced sensitivity to somatic pain (Bouin, Meunier, Riberdy-Poitras, & Poitras, 2001; Verne, Robinson, & Price, 2001). The discrepancies in these findings are likely due to methodological factors and potential differences in patient selection.

Numerous studies indicate increased psychological distress among patients with IBS compared to healthy controls. For example, scores on instruments assessing depression and anxiety are higher among IBS patients compared to healthy individuals and to patients with headache (Blanchard & Scharff, 2002). In addition, psychiatric disorders, especially anxiety and depressive disorders, are more common among IBS patients than healthy controls (Whitehead et al., 2002; Mayer, Craske, & Naliboff, 2001). Also, stress has been identified as an exacerbating factor in IBS. For example, IBS patients reported higher levels of life stress than both controls and individuals with abdominal pain not due to IBS, and stress predicted subsequent bowel symptoms more strongly among IBS patients than the other two groups (Whitehead, Crowell, Robinson, Heller, & Schuster, 1992). By comparing individuals who meet diagnostic criteria for IBS but have not sought treatment (i.e., IBS nonpatients) to patients recruited in the clinical setting (IBS patients), investigators have reported that psychological factors, including mood disturbance, abuse history, and psychosocial stress predict health care seeking among patients with IBS (Koloski, Talley, & Boyce, 2001). Psychosocial factors are also associated with increased symptom severity and poorer quality of life in IBS (Naliboff, Balice, & Mayer, 1998; Drossman, 1999).

Whether psychological factors are involved in the development of IBS or simply result from the disorder has not been determined. However, recent investigations of the development of postinfectious IBS following acute gastroenteritis provide some information in this regard. Gwee and colleagues (1996, 1999) administered psychometric instruments to patients hospitalized during episodes of acute gastroenteritis and followed them to investigate the development of post-infectious IBS. Their findings indicate that psychological measures, including recent stressful life events and a measure of hypochondriasis, were significantly higher in patients who went on to develop IBS versus those who did not. These findings are intriguing, but they may reflect patients' psychological response to the acute gastroenteritis. Also, whether the results are generalizable to patients with IBS not associated with gastroenteritis is not known.

Psychological treatments are successful in ameliorating the symptoms of IBS. Randomized controlled trials support the effectiveness of brief psychodynamic psychotherapy, hypnotherapy, and cognitive-behavioral therapy in the treatment of IBS, though CBT seemed somewhat less consistent in its effects (Blanchard & Scharff, 2002). Recently, the effectiveness of brief psychotherapy was compared to the SSRI paroxetine in the treatment of IBS. Both treatment conditions were similar in their effectiveness and were superior to standard care in improving health-related quality of life, but only the psychotherapy treatment was associated with a significant reduction in health care costs over the ensuing year (Creed et al., 2003). However, a more recent controlled trial reported no advantage for relaxation or cognitive-behavioral therapy over standard medical care for IBS, as all three groups demonstrated considerable improvement (Boyce, Talley, Balaam, Koloski, & Truman, 2003). Taken together, these findings suggest that psychological treatments, especially hypnosis and brief psychodynamic therapy, are effective in the management of IBS.

language: Given the subjective nature of pain, as it is now defined, and the heavy reliance on verbal reporting to assess pain, the language used by individuals to communicate their pain is an important issue. Several pain-assessment instruments rely on the use of verbal descriptors of pain (*see* MCGILL PAIN QUESTIONNAIRE and PAIN ASSESSMENT), and the use of such descriptors is influenced by the meaning ascribed to them (i.e., the pain language). Indeed, individuals from different clinical groups (e.g., students versus patients) and from different cultures use verbal descriptors of pain differently (Tammaro, Berggren, & Bergenholtz, 1997; Moore, Brodsgaard, Miller, Mao, & Dworkin, 1997). Moreover, some findings indicate that pain patients from different diagnostic groups use different verbal descriptors to describe their pain (Kramer, Harker, & Wong, 2002; Mauro, Tagliaferro, Montini, & Zanolla, 2001). One of the most carefully developed instruments which assesses pain via pain language is the Multidimensional Affect and Pain Survey (MAPS) developed by Clark, Fletcher, Janal, & Carroll (1995). The MAPS consists of 101 verbal descriptors of pain and emotion retained from an original list of 270 words through iterative empirical validation (Clark et al., 1995, 2003). The MAPS verbal descriptors are mathematically partitioned into three major categories: somatosensory pain, emotional pain, and well-being, and multiple subscales (or subclusters) are within each major category. The MAPS provides a well-validated instrument that assesses multiple dimensions of pain, distress, and well-being.

learning: *See* BEHAVIORAL FACTORS.

legal issues: A variety of legal issues is relevant to the field of pain management. First, patients whose pain results from personal injury or work-related trauma often retain legal counsel. Many clinicians believe that pending litigation is associated with poorer prognosis and an unfavorable response to treatment, and some evidence supports this contention. For example, the presence of litigation or disability compensation predicts poorer outcomes following spine surgery for back pain (Epker & Block, 2001). Also, some evidence suggests that patients receiving compensation report more severe symptomatology and exhibit poorer response to rehabilitation (Rainville, Sobel, Hartigan, & Wright, 1997; Tollison, Satterthwaite, Kriegel, & Hinnant, 1990). Policy changes have also been associated with pain-related outcomes. For example Saskatchewan, Canada, removed payments for pain and suffering from their tort-compensation system for traffic injuries, and subsequently, the incidence of claims and the duration from date of injury to claim closure were significantly reduced for both whiplash and low back pain (Cassidy, Carroll, Cote, Berglund, & Nygren, 2003; Cassidy et al., 2000). These findings suggest that legal issues can be associated with pain-related outcomes, but the mechanisms underlying these associations remain unclear. Given this medicolegal context, pain psychologists are increasingly called upon to perform evaluation and to provide expert testimony regarding the extent of patients' psychological injury and disability, and psychologists should represent their expertise accurately and testify only within their expertise (Main, 1999).

Additional legal issues that should be mentioned include regulatory issues surrounding the prescription of controlled substances, about which physicians are often concerned (Zacny et al., 2003). In addition, there can be liability for inadequate pain treatment. These legal issues related to pain treatment should be understood by providers involved in the delivery of pain management.

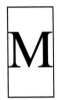 **malingering:** Malingering refers to the intentional production or exaggeration of symptoms motivated by external incentives (e.g., financial compensation, obtaining drugs) (American Psychiatric Association, 1994). Malingering has also been referred to as *compensation neurosis*. The nature of pain as a subjective complaint makes it difficult to detect malingering, since no medical tests are available that can detect the presence (or absence) of pain. Also, factitious disorder, conversion disorder, and other somatoform disorders are difficult to distinguish from malingering. Thus, good evidence on the prevalence of malingering in chronic pain populations is unavailable. In a review of the topic, Fishbain, Cutler, Rosomoff, & Rosomoff (1999) note that malingering among pain patients appears to be rare, though many providers believe the frequency is high.

Several signs and symptoms are often interpreted as representative of malingering. For example, patients who are inconsistent in their presentation, such as verbal reports of severe pain in the absence of overt pain behavior, may be suspected of malingering. Several studies suggest that instructing healthy controls or medical patients to simulate (i.e., feign) chronic pain when responding to questionnaires results in much higher than typical elevations on clinical scales of psychological distress and pain-related symptoms (McGuire & Shores, 2001; McGuire, Harvey, & Shores, 2001). Also, validity scales on some psychometric instruments are thought to detect a "fake-bad" response set, though the false positive rate is quite high (Butcher, Arbisi, Atlis, & McNulty, 2003). These types of data are often interpreted as reflecting malingering, but no evidence shows that these methods are valid as tests of malingering (Fishbain et al., 1999). As previously discussed (*see* FUNCTIONAL ASSESSMENT), measures of variability on performance-based functional testing were initially touted as useful in detecting malingering, though the data do not support that claim (Fishbain et al., 1999; Robinson & Dannecker, 2004).

Although malingering undoubtedly does occur in the chronic pain setting, presently no reliable and valid method is available for detecting malingering. Moreover, many of the signs and symptoms thought to reflect malingering are nonspecific and can be produced by numerous factors. Additional research is needed to improve our ability to detect malingering.

McGill Pain Questionnaire: The McGill Pain Questionnaire (MPQ) is among the most widely used pain-measurement tools in existence. It was originally developed by Melzack and Torgerson (1971) at McGill University. These investigators first identified 102 words related to pain from the clinical literature, and they asked physicians and other volunteers to place the words in small groups that described different aspects of the pain experience. The words were categorized into three major classes: (1) sensory words, (2) affective words, and (3) evaluative words. Within these major categories, words were then further divided into smaller subgroups of words that were qualitatively similar. Next, groups of physicians, patients, and students were asked to assign a numerical value to each word based on the intensity of pain that the word implied, and the words in each subgroup were then rank-ordered according to these numerical weights. In administering the resultant questionnaire to patients, it was determined that additional descriptors were needed; therefore, four additional subgroups of descriptors were added, which comprise the miscellaneous subscale of the MPQ. The final questionnaire includes 20 groups of two to six words and yields four subscale scores computed by summing the rank values of the highest endorsed word in each subgroup of that scale: sensory, affective, evaluative, and miscellaneous (Melzack, 1975). A total score (Pain Rating Index) is derived by summing the highest rank values of all subgroups. Also, the Present Pain Intensity (PPI) is the patient ratings of pain, ranging from none (0) to excruciating (5). A short form of the MPQ has also been developed, which appears to correlate well with the original (Melzack, 1987).

Considerable evidence has accrued supporting the reliability and validity of the MPQ, and it has been found sensitive to treatment-related changes in pain (Melzack & Katz, 2001). Also, the MPQ has useful discriminative capacity as patients with different forms of clinical pain endorse different patterns of descriptors (Melzack & Katz, 2001), though some findings suggest that the discriminant validity of the McGill subscales is inadequate due to high intercorrelations among the scales (Turk, Rudy, & Salovey, 1985). Some evidence questions the factor structure of the MPQ as well as the validity and reliability of some of the descriptors (Clark et al., 2003; Fernandez & Boyle, 2001). These concerns notwithstanding, the MPQ remains an extremely widely used instrument, and it has the distinct advantage of providing valuable qualitative information regarding patients' pain experiences.

memory for pain: Memory for pain is an important issue, since assessment of patients' pain and determination of treatment outcome are based largely on patients' memory of their pain. The literature is inconsistent regarding how accurate one's memory for pain is; some studies indicate reasonable accuracy, while others report either under- or overreporting of pain (Erskine, Morley, & Pearce, 1990). As one might expect, time can adversely impact the accuracy of memory for pain. For example, patients with low back pain were asked to recall the number of pain-free days they had experienced in the past week, month, and six months, and these retrospective reports were compared to daily diary data (McGorry, Webster, Snook, & Hsiang, 1999). One-week and one-month recall was accurate; however, recall over the past six months was significantly different from the diary data. Twenty percent of patients overestimated the number of days in pain, 58 percent underestimated their pain, and 22 percent were accurate. Women were more accurate than men, and patients with recurrent pain tended to recall more accurately than those with chronic pain. In another study, Everts and colleagues (1999) reported that patients who had experienced chest pain recalled higher levels of pain six months after hospitalization than they reported at the time of the episode. This overestimation of pain was particularly characteristic of patients with high levels of emotional distress. This association between emotional distress and pain recall has also been observed for experimental pain. Specifically, healthy subjects reported their pain during a cold-pressor procedure and were called one-week and 18 months later and queried regarding their pain recall (Gedney, Logan, & Baron, 2003). One-week recall of pain intensity was most strongly associated with actual pain intensity during the procedure;

however, 18-month recall of pain intensity and recall of pain unpleasantness at both time points were best predicted by the state anxiety
that the subject reported prior to the cold pressor procedure. Thus, affective state at the time of the pain experience was the best predictor
of long-term pain recall.

Several studies in the acute-pain setting demonstrate the peak-end
phenomenon, which refers to the finding that recall of pain is based
on two factors: (1) the peak pain experienced during the episode or
procedure, and (2) the pain experienced at the end of the episode. For
example, patients undergoing colonoscopy and lithotripsy provided
real-time pain ratings during the procedure and were asked to retrospectively rate the total amount of pain experienced during the procedure within an hour of its termination (Redelmeier & Kahneman,
1996). Patients' retrospective pain reports were strongly correlated
with peak pain and end pain, but not with the duration of the procedure. In a subsequent intervention study based on these findings, patients undergoing colonoscopy were randomly assigned to standard
protocol or an extended duration condition in which the colonoscope
remained quiescently placed in the rectum for three minutes at the
end of the procedure (Redelmeier, Katz, & Kahneman, 2003). This
intervention was designed to reduce the "end pain," thereby decreasing the amount of recalled pain. The results indicated that the ex-
tended-treatment patients rated the procedure as less aversive and
showed a higher rate of returning for repeated colonoscopies over the
follow-up period. The peak-end phenomenon has also been reported
among patients with rheumatoid arthritis, suggesting that this phenomenon also occurs in chronic pain (Stone, Broderick, Kaell, Deles-
Paul, & Porter, 2000).

These findings illustrate the potential for bias in pain recall and
demonstrate the multiple factors that affect memory for pain. These
issues should be considered when evaluating patients' clinical pain
and determining treatment efficacy based on retrospective reporting.

menstrual cycle: Epidemiological and survey data indicate that
more than one-third of women in the general population experience
significant physical and psychological symptoms across the menstrual cycle, with pain being among the most common symptoms
(Huerta-Franco & Malacara, 1993; Kessel & Coppen, 1963). Also,
some pain disorders show menstrual-cycle related exacerbations, and

pain is a common symptom in several menstrual-cycle disorders (e.g., dysmenorrhea, menstrual migraine, premenstrual syndrome). Multiple studies examined menstrual cycle influences on responses to experimentally induced pain in humans. Although the findings are somewhat mixed, a recent qualitative review (Fillingim & Ness, 2000) and a meta-analysis (Riley, Robinson, Wise, & Price, 1999) both concluded that for most forms of painful stimulation (with the exception of electrical stimulation), higher pain thresholds and tolerances were reported during the follicular compared to periovulatory and luteal and perimenstrual phases. The meta-analysis indicated that the effect sizes were small to moderate (Riley et al., 1999). Taken together, these findings indicate that the experience of pain varies across the menstrual cycle, and that hormonal fluctuations are important to consider in the evaluation and management of women's pain.

mindfulness-based stress reduction: Mindfulness-based stress reduction (MBSR) is a stress management and relaxation intervention based on mindfulness meditation, which derives from Buddhist traditions and emphasizes moment-to-moment awareness of life and its experiences (Kabat-Zinn, 1990). MBSR has attracted tremendous interest in the past 20 years and has been applied to a wide range of psychological and medical conditions, though the quality and quantity of empirical support for MBSR has been questioned (Bishop, 2002). Two more recent controlled trials provide evidence that MBSR reduces psychological and physical symptomatology in community-based samples and in medical patient populations (Reibel, Greeson, Brainard, & Rosenzweig, 2001; Williams, Kolar, Reger, & Pearson, 2001). The earliest published reports of MBSR were based on treatment of patients with chronic pain. In an uncontrolled study, MBSR produced significant reductions in pain and other medical symptoms and in psychological distress in a heterogeneous sample of 51 chronic pain patients (Kabat-Zinn, 1982). Subsequently, MBSR was provided to 90 pain patients, and significant reductions in pain, emotional distress, and medication use, and increases in activity levels occurred, while no such improvements were observed in a comparison group of patients receiving standard medical care (Kabat-Zinn, Lipworth, & Burney, 1985). In a recent randomized controlled trial, an intervention that included mindfulness meditation and Qigong movement therapy was no more effective than an education control condition for patients with fibromyalgia MBSR (Astin et al., 2003). Taken together, the findings suggest that MBSR may be helpful in reducing physical and psychological symptoms; however, additional controlled trials are needed to determine the effectiveness of MBSR for patients with chronic pain.

Minnesota Multiphasic Personality Inventory: The Minnesota Multiphasic Personality Inventory (MMPI) is the most widely used psychological instrument used in the clinical assessment of patients with chronic pain. The original MMPI included 566 true-false items, which yielded three validity scales and ten clinical scales, reflecting the patient's level of psychological disturbance. The original test was first published in 1943 (Hathaway & McKinley, 1943), and the revised version, the MMPI-2, was published in 1989 (Butcher, Dahlstrom, Graham, Tellegen, & Kaemmer, 1989). One major improvement in the MMPI-2 was the inclusion of a more representative normative sample (Butcher et al., 1989). It is important to recognize that the standardization samples for the MMPI and MMPI-2 did not include medical patients; therefore, elevations on clinical scales may reflect medical symptoms in patients with chronic physical conditions rather than psychological disturbance (Bradley & McKendree-Smith, 2001).

A vast amount of research has been conducted utilizing the MMPI and MMPI-2 in chronic pain populations. Cluster analyses were used to identify MMPI and MMPI-2 profile patterns in chronic pain patients, and these studies produced three or four profile types (Bradley & McKendree-Smith, 2001). The three-cluster solutions included: (1) a group of patients with elevations on the "neurotic triad" scales (hypochondriasis, depression, hysteria), who displayed high levels of pain and affective distress; (2) a group of patients with high scores across multiple clinical scales, which reflected high levels of psychopathology and substantial social dysfunction; and (3) a profile with no significant clinical elevations, who showed relatively minimal psychological disturbance. One group of investigators, in addition to these profiles, identified a cluster characterized by elevations on the hypochondriasis and hysteria scales but not on depression (i.e., a "conversion V") (Costello, Hulsey, Schoenfeld, & Ramamurthy, 1987). Limited evidence suggests that certain profile types may respond more poorly to treatment, though evidence to the contrary also exists (see Bradley & McKendree-Smith, 2001, for a review).

Other studies examined the utility of individual MMPI scales in predicting prognosis among patients with chronic pain. For example, numerous studies reported that elevations of certain MMPI scales (especially scales 1 and 3) predict poor outcomes from surgical intervention (Burchiel et al., 1995; Uomoto, Turner, & Herron, 1988; Turner, Herron, & Weiner, 1986). Moreover, in a large prospective study of industrial workers, scale 3 (Hysteria) of the MMPI was one of the two factors that best predicted which individuals would file a claim for work-related back injury (Bigos et al., 1992). Another study administered the MMPI to patients presenting with acute low back pain, and scale 3 was a significant predictor of failure to return to work at the six-month follow-up (Gatchel, Polatin, & Kinney, 1995). These findings demonstrate the clinical utility of the MMPI and MMPI-2 in chronic pain populations.

motivation: In recent years, motivational factors have received increased attention as important mediators of treatment outcome. Multiple theories of motivation exist, including physiologically based theories (e.g., drive reduction), personality-based theories (e.g., Maslow's hierarchy of needs), cognitive theories (e.g., self-efficacy), and behavioral theories (e.g., operant conditioning). Each theory attempts to explain the cessation, initiation, and/or maintenance of behavior.

One approach to investigating the importance of motivational factors in pain has been to manipulate motivation in studies of experimental and clinical pain. Regarding the former, Cabanac (1986) provided a monetary incentive and found that subjects' pain tolerance times increased linearly in relation to the logarithm of the amount of payment they received, suggesting that the money served as a motivational factor that influenced pain tolerance performance. In another experiment, Baker and Kirsch (1991) found that both instruction in cognitive coping and monetary incentive increased pain tolerance. The monetary incentive was more effective, but the two strategies combined produced additive effects. In another study, subjects' pain tolerance increased when they were given specific quotas or goals to achieve, but the addition of monetary reinforcement did not produce an incremental effect (Dolce et al., 1986). Thus, both monetary and goal-based incentives can increase pain tolerance, though a recent study reported no effect of incentive on pain tolerance (Lowery, Fillingim, & Wright, 2003).

Motivation is relevant to clinical pain management in that treatment often requires that patients alter their behavior (e.g., change medication use, increase activity, implement new coping skills) and maintain this behavior change over an extended period of time. Moreover, there may be competing incentives for some patients (e.g., the desire to improve physical function versus the desire to avoid pain). Jensen, Nielson, & Kerns (2003) recently proposed a motivational model of pain self-management that incorporates aspects of multiple theories of motivation and behavior change. This model proposes that patients will change their pain self-management behavior only after they reach a certain stage of readiness to change (*see* STAGES OF CHANGE). Readiness to change is determined by: (1) the perceived importance of the behavior change, and (2) patients' self-efficacy for successfully accomplishing the behavior change (*see* SELF-EFFICACY).

The authors discuss several treatment implications of this model. First, clinicians should attempt to create positive expectancies and reduce negative expectancies regarding the outcome of self-management behaviors, as this will enhance the perceived importance of the behavior change. Also, changing the contingencies for patients' pain-management behaviors is recommended. Specifically, it is important to reinforce adaptive self-management behaviors (e.g., increased activity, use of coping skills) and removing reinforcers for maladaptive strategies (e.g., activity avoidance, catastrophizing). In addition, increasing patients' self-efficacy for pain self-management is an important component of treatment (*see* SELF-EFFICACY).

Motivational interviewing represents an intervention designed to enhance motivation for behavior change, and its application to the treatment of chronic pain has recently been discussed (Jensen, 2002). The purpose of motivational interviewing is to address and resolve patients' ambivalence toward implementing therapeutic behavior change. The five principles of motivational interviewing are: (1) express empathy; (2) develop discrepancy between patients' current behavior and their goals; (3) avoid argumentation, as this can increase resistance; (4) roll with resistance through reframing patients' concerns; and (5) support self-efficacy (Miller & Rollnick, 2002). Although motivational interviewing has been successfully applied to behavior change in other clinical populations, presently no empirical data exists regarding its effectiveness in the treatment of chronic pain. Nonetheless, motivational factors are undoubtedly important in chronic pain management, and future research to determine the efficacy of motivational interventions in clinical pain treatment is needed.

Multidimensional Pain Inventory: The Multidimensional Pain Inventory (MPI) was originally developed as the West Haven-Yale Multidimensional Pain Inventory (WHYMPI) by Kerns, Turk, & Rudy (1985). This questionnaire, designed to broadly assess pain-related adjustment, included three sections that would assess: (1) the impact of pain on the patient's life; (2) how significant others respond to the patient's pain; and (3) the patient's participation in various daily activities. Numerous studies demonstrated that the MPI has good psychometric qualities (see Bradley & McKendree-Smith, 2001, for a review). Turk and Rudy (1988) performed cluster analysis of the MPI in a heterogeneous chronic pain population, which revealed three profiles: (1) *dysfunctional*—characterized by high pain severity, interference, and emotional distress along with low-perceived life control and general activity levels; (2) *interpersonally distressed*—characterized by low-perceived social support and reports that significant others are punishing in their response to the patient's pain; and (3) *adaptive copers*—characterized by low levels of pain, interference, and affective distress, and high levels of perceived life control and general activity. These clusters were replicated numerous times in other samples, including patients with fibromyalgia, temporomandibular disorders, and headache (Jamison, Rudy, Penzien, & Mosley Jr., 1994; Rudy, Turk, Zaki, & Curtin, 1989; Turk, Okifuji, Sinclair, & Starz, 1996; Turk & Rudy, 1990; Walter & Brannon, 1991).

The profile classifications were supposed to be used to tailor treatment; however, this has received limited direct empirical attention. Some studies found that patients with all three MPI profile classifications benefit equally from multidisciplinary treatment (Gatchel et al., 2002; Bergstrom, Jensen, Bodin, Linton, & Nygren, 2001), and one study surprisingly reported that dysfunctional patients showed greater benefit from multimodal treatment than did the other two profile types (Rudy, Turk, Kubinski, & Zaki, 1995). One clinical trial compared standard multidisciplinary treatment to multidisciplinary treatment plus a tailored cognitive therapy component for temporomandibular disorder with dysfunctional profiles (Turk, Rudy, Kubinski, Zaki, & Greco, 1996). Although patients undergoing both treatments showed improvement, only those in the tailored protocol maintained their improvements at the six-month follow-up.

The MPI is a valuable tool, as it assesses multiple aspects of pain-related adjustment and yields three relatively stable profile types. Whether treatment tailoring on the basis of profile type will significantly improve outcomes has not been determined.

 neuromatrix: Melzack (1999, 1996) introduced the neuromatrix theory of pain as a sequel to the gate control theory of pain (Melzack & Wall, 1965). The neuromatrix theory proposes that the neuromatrix is a widely distributed neural network in the brain, including thalamic, cortical, and limbic components, and this serves as the neuroanatomical substrate for sensory experience. The architecture of the neuromatrix is determined by both genetic influences and sensory inputs. The neuromatirx continuously outputs a neurosignature, which is responsible for our sensory experience, including pain. This neurosignature is influenced by multiple factors, including tonic somatic input, phasic sensory input, attention, mood, past experience, and numerous physiological systems (e.g., opioid system, immune system, endocrine system). The overall message of the neuromatrix theory is that the experience of pain is actively sculpted by multiple internal and external influences, and dispositional and situational psychological factors contribute heavily to the neural substrate of pain.

neuropathic pain: Neuropathic pain refers to "pain initiated or caused by a primary lesion or dysfunction in the nervous system" (Merskey & Bogduk, 1994, p. 212). The involved nerve(s) can be located in the central or the peripheral nervous system. Three common types of neuropathic pain have been identified: peripheral neuropathic pain (e.g., painful diabetic neuropathy, postherpetic neuralgia); central neuropathic pain (e.g., central poststroke pain, spinal cord injury pain); and cancer-associated neuropathic pain (e.g., postmastectomy pain, chemotherapy-induced polyneuropathy) (Dworkin, Nagasako, & Galer, 2001). Patients with neuropathic pain frequently choose sensory adjectives (e.g., burning, tingling, cold, pricking) and less frequently choose affective words (e.g., fearful) on the McGill Pain Questionnaire to describe their pain compared to patients with nonneuropathic pain (Boureau, Doubrere, & Luu, 1990). Conducting mechanism-based diagnosis of neuropathic pain (Woolf & Max, 2001) typically requires the use of quantitative sensory testing (QST, *see* PSYCHOPHYSICS). For example, Pappagallo, Oaklander, Quatrano-Piacentini, Clark, & Raja (2000) conducted QST in patients with postherpetic neuralgia and noted different patterns of sensory disturbance in subgroups of patients, suggesting different underlying mechanisms. Similarly, patients with complex regional pain syndrome, another neuropathic pain condition, were classified as having localized (i.e., restricted to the affected limb) versus generalized (i.e., extending well beyond the affected area) sensory impairments based on standard neurological examination (Rommel, Malin, Zenz, & Janig, 2001). Then, more sophisticated QST was performed, which revealed a different pattern of perceptual abnormalities in the two groups. Specifically, patients with generalized sensory impairment showed more extensive sensory deficits compared to the localized patients. However, the generalized impairment patients also showed a higher frequency of mechanical allodynia. It is hoped that mechanism-based diagnosis, including the use of QST, to determine the underlying pathophysiology contributing to neuropathic pain will inform pain treatment and enhance clinical outcomes.

neuropsychological testing: Neuropsychological testing refers to the use of psychometric measures to assess neurocognitive function, including memory, motor function, executive function, and other cognitive processes. Patients with chronic pain frequently report cognitive deficits, including forgetfulness, minor accidents, difficulty completing tasks, and difficulties with attention (McCracken & Iverson, 2001; Suhr, 2003). Numerous studies have examined neuropsychological function among patients with chronic pain, and evidence shows that patients with chronic pain perform more poorly on neuropsychological tests compared to healthy controls (Hart, Wade, & Martelli, 2003; Hart, Martelli, & Zasler, 2000; Kessels, Aleman, Verhagen, & van Luijtelaar, 2000). The reasons for these deficits are not fully understood; however, emotional distress, psychological stress, and neuroendocrine function have been associated with cognitive performance in pain populations (Sephton et al., 2003; Hart et al., 2003; Suhr, 2003; Iezzi, Archibald, Barnett, Klinck, & Duckworth, 1999). Sleep disturbance could also contribute. The use of centrally acting medications, especially opioids, can adversely affect neurocognitive function. Studies in healthy volunteers report that acute administration of opioids impairs neuropsychological performance (Schneider et al., 1999; Cleeland et al., 1996); however, it seems likely that long-term administration of these medications to patients with moderate to severe clinical pain could produce substantially different cognitive effects. Indeed, several recent studies indicate that long-term opioid therapy actually tends to improve neurocognitive performance among patients with chronic pain, perhaps due to the improved pain control afforded by the medication (Tassain et al., 2003; Jamison et al., 2003). Taken together, these findings suggest that patients with chronic pain show cognitive deficits compared to controls, and while the reasons for this are not completely understood, pain-related sequelae such as affective distress and psychosocial stress are likely contributors.

neuroticism: Neuroticism refers to a personality dimension characterized by emotional lability, nervousness, and the tendency to worry. Several personality instruments are available to assess neuroticism. For example, the first three clinical scales of the MMPI (hypochondriasis, depression, and hysteria) are often referred to as the *neurotic triad,* and previous studies demonstrate significant elevations on these scales in a significant proportion of chronic pain patients (*see* MINNESOTA MULTIPHASIC PERSONALITY INVENTORY). Also, in studies of chronic pain patients using an instrument that measures neuroticism directly, neuroticism has associated with the affective dimensions of pain (i.e., pain unpleasantness, pain-related suffering, and illness behavior), but not the sensory dimension (Harkins, Price, & Braith, 1989; Wade, Dougherty, Hart, Rafii, & Price, 1992). Recent evidence suggests that neuroticism may moderate the association between pain severity and catastrophizing, such that high neuroticism is associated with greater catastrophizing at lower levels of pain (Goubert, Crombez, & Van Damme, 2004). Thus, it seems likely that personality characteristics associated with neuroticism (e.g., negative affectivity, anxiety, hypervigilance) may influence primarily the reporting and appraisal of pain rather than the sensory experience.

nocebo: The term nocebo is the opposite of the placebo response. Specifically, the nocebo response refers to an exacerbation of symptoms following administration of a treatment that the patient believes will make him or her worse. The nocebo response appears to be mediated by expectancies, such that patients experience increased pain because they expect it. In one study of the nocebo phenomenon, thoracotomy patients were administered saline in a hidden fashion or they received saline with the instruction that it would cause an increase in their pain within 30 minutes (nocebo instructions) (Benedetti, Amanzio, Casadio, Oliaro, & Maggi, 1997). The nocebo group reported a substantial increase in pain, and the hidden injection produced no change. Moreover, when the cholecystokinin (CCK) receptor antagonist proglumide was administered, the nocebo effect was abolished. This indicates that not only do negative expectancies adversely affect pain, but that they do so through a specific neurochemical mechanism (i.e., by activating CCK receptors). Such nocebo effects may also contribute significantly to the experience of medication-related side effects (Barsky, Saintfort, Rogers, & Borus, 2002). The nocebo effect has important implications for treating patients with chronic pain. Many patients have had multiple unsuccessful past treatments, which can generate negative expectancies; therefore, the treatment process needs to include replacing these negative expectancies with positive ones.

nociception: Nociception refers to activation of nociceptors, which are receptors "preferentially sensitive to a noxious (i.e., tissue damaging) stimulus or a stimulus which would become noxious if prolonged" (Merskey & Bogduk, 1994, p. 213). Thus, nociception is the most peripheral segment of the neural responses that often contribute to the experience of pain. Nociception can occur in the absence of pain and pain can occur in the absence of nociception. Thus, use of the term "pain receptor" or "pain fiber" is ill-advised.

nonorganic signs: *See* WADDELL SIGNS.

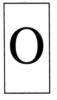

obstetric pain: Labor and delivery are almost universally painful, and many women report or expect this to be among the most painful experiences of their lives (Robinson et al., 2003; Melzack, Taenzer, Feldman, & Kinch, 1981). Numerous pharmacologic and nonpharmacologic techniques are effective for controlling the pain of childbirth (Lee-man, Fontaine, King, Klein, & Ratcliffe, 2000a, 2003b). Nonetheless, pain during childbirth is a significant predictor of appraising childbirth as traumatic (Soet, Brack, & DiIorio, 2003), and fear of childbirth pain is quite common among pregnant women (Geiss-buehler & Eberhard, 2002). Evidence in animals and humans demonstrates pregnancy-induced analgesia—a decrease in pain sensitivity that is produced by the hormonal and biological changes that accompany pregnancy (Gintzler & Liu, 2000). However, the findings of Saisto, Kaaja, Ylikorkala, & Halmesmaki (2001) suggest that fear may influence pain perception in pregnancy, as women with fear of labor showed significantly lower pain tolerance and higher ratings of cold-pressor pain compared to women with no fear of labor. Desirability of pregnancy is correlated with lower pain, and women use multiple coping strategies to manage pain during childbirth (Dannen-bring, Stevens, & House, 1997; Niven & Gijsbers, 1996).

operant conditioning: *See* BEHAVIORAL FACTORS.

opioid therapy: In the 1970s and 1980s, the era of behaviorally based multidisciplinary pain treatment, one goal of therapy was to decrease patients' use of opioids. From a behavioral perspective, opioid consumption was conceptualized as a maladaptive pain behavior that produced primarily negative effects on the patient (e.g., depression, side effects, psychological and physical dependence) (Fordyce, 1976). Indeed, the use of the pain cocktail was recommended, which involved administering the patient's medications in time-contingent basis using a flavored liquid, and the opioid dose was gradually decreased to zero (Fordyce, 1976). In recent years, the zeitgeist has changed dramatically, such that opioid therapy for chronic noncancer pain is now widely used. Indeed, medical prescriptions for opioids have increased dramatically during the 1990s (Joranson, Ryan, Gilson, & Dahl, 2000; Zacny et al., 2003). The use of chronic opioid therapy for chronic noncancer pain remains a hotly debated issue among pain clinicians, and several issues must be considered when discussing chronic opioid therapy.

To determine the utility of opioid therapy, a cost-benefit analysis is most appropriate. Regarding costs, one obvious concern is addiction, which was discussed previously (*see* ADDICTION). The other major costs are adverse effects, the most common being sedation and cognitive impairment, nausea/vomiting, respiratory depression, and constipation (Nicholson, 2003). Constipation is typically managed with laxatives and stool softeners, and nausea/vomiting usually habituate and can be managed medically in many patients. Tolerance to the sedating effects of opioids generally occurs rapidly, and as previously discussed (see NEUROPSYCHOLOGICAL TESTING), the evidence does not indicate significant cognitive impairment with opioids. Respiratory depression, although potentially dangerous, can typically be managed through careful dose titration, and patients usually show tolerance to this side effect (Nicholson, 2003). Although opioid side effects are often transitory and clinically manageable, it is important to recognize that many patients discontinue opioid therapy due to side effects. For example, in a recent controlled study of oxycodone in patients with arthritis, 43 of 88 patients in the two active drug conditions discontinued therapy due to ineffective treatment or adverse effects (Roth et al., 2000). In another controlled trial using time-released morphine, 11 of 61 patients dropped out of the study during morphine titration (Moulin et al., 1996), and 52 percent of patients discontinued a trial of codeine due to adverse effects or insufficient pain relief (Kjaersgaard-Andersen et al., 1990). Thus, in a substantial proportion of patients with chronic noncancer pain, opioids produce inadequate pain relief and/or unacceptable adverse effects.

Regarding the benefits of opioid therapy, an important, yet often overlooked issue is the effectiveness of opioids for chronic pain. Numerous cross-sectional studies conducted in multidisciplinary pain treatment settings indicate that opioid use among patients with chronic noncancer pain is associated with greater pain and functional impairment and poorer treatment response (Buckley, Sizemore, & Charlton, 1986; Maruta & Swanson, 1981; Maruta, Swanson, & Finlayson, 1979; Turner, Calsyn, Fordyce, & Ready, 1982). A survey of patients with spinal pain, ranging from acute to chronic pain, indicated that those treated with opioids had greater pain and poorer physical and social function than those not treated with opioids (Fanciullo et al., 2002). However, these findings are likely based on patient populations who failed previous medical and surgical treatments, which may offer a negatively biased view of opioid treatment. Several controlled and uncontrolled clinical trials of opioid therapy for chronic noncancer pain have been conducted, and two recent reviews of these findings concluded that opioids are generally effective for chronic noncancer pain, especially for carefully selected patients with nociceptive pain (Collett, 2001; Graven, de Vet, van Kleef, & Weber, 2000). However, these optimistic reports regarding the effectiveness of opioids are often based on the subset of patients who complete treatment, which may overestimate efficacy.

Additional costs of opioid therapy that are less frequently considered include the effects on gonadal hormones and the possibility of opioid-induced hyperalgesia. Several clinical studies demonstrated that chronic opioid use produces dysfunction in the gonadal hormonal axis, which is associated with decreased libido and reduced energy among patients (Abs et al., 2000; Daniell, 2002a, 2000b; Finch, Roberts, Price, Hadlow, & Pullan, 2000; Roberts, Finch, Pullan, Bhagat, & Price, 2002). Also, a substantial basic science literature suggests that sustained opioid exposure can produce central nervous system alterations that enhance sensitivity to pain, which is known as opioid-induced hyperalgesia (Mao, 2002; Ossipov, Lai, Vanderah, & Porreca, 2003). This has not been carefully studied in humans, but evidence indicates that opioid abusers are more sensitive to experimental pain compared to healthy controls (Compton, Charuvastra, & Ling, 2001). The potential consequences of opioid therapy merit further clinical investigation.

When the data are examined closely, the magnitude of the effects in placebo-controlled trials is somewhat underwhelming. For example, in one of the most well-designed trials, Moulin and colleagues (1996) examined the efficacy of oral morphine for treatment of chronic musculoskeletal pain in patients who had failed to respond to nonopioid analgesics. The protocol was a randomized, double-blind, crossover design, and patients also received concurrent cognitive-behavioral treatment. Each treatment period included a two-week washout phase, a three-week titration phase, and a six-week evaluation phase. Of the 61 patients who initiated treatment, 15 dropped out due to side effects or inadequate pain relief (11 during morphine titration and four during placebo titration), such that 46 patients completed the study. For the patients who received morphine first, mean pain intensity decreased from approximately 7.8 to 6.8 on a ten-point visual analog scale. The placebo-first group showed no change in pain. Interestingly, when the two groups crossed over, the morphine-first group maintained their pain reduction through the placebo phase, and the placebo-first group failed to respond to morphine. Also, no differences were observed between morphine and placebo conditions for depression, anxiety, disability, or health-related quality of life.

Other controlled studies suggest similarly modest magnitudes of pain relief. For example, Jamison and colleagues compared the effects of naproxen to standard opioid dosing and dosing titrated to effect (Jamison, Raymond, Slawsby, Nedeljkovic, & Katz, 1998). During the treatment phase, the average pain levels were 66.5, 59.8, and 54.9 (on a 0 to 100 scale) for the naproxen, standard opioid dose, and titrated opioid dose conditions, respectively. In another trial involving arthritis pain, 40 mg controlled release (CR) oxycodone decreased pain from 2.5 to 1.5, on a four-point categorical scale (0 = none, 1 = mild, 2 = moderate, 3 = severe), while 20 mg CR oxycodone reduced pain from 2.5 to 2 and placebo reduce pain from 2.4 to 2.1 (Roth et al., 2000). In another recent arthritis trial, different forms of extended-release morphine produced a 22 to 26 percent reduction in arthritis pain compared to a 14 percent reduction with placebo (Caldwell et al., 2002).

One misconception regarding opioid treatment is that neuropathic pain is opioid-resistant. Two recent clinical trials demonstrate the efficacy of opioid therapy for neuropathic pain, and the magnitude of the effect appears larger than that typically seen for nociceptive pain (Raja et al., 2002; Rowbotham et al., 2003). Also, in a recent trial, a greater proportion of patients with neuropathic pain (41 percent) were morphine responders compared to patients with nociceptive pain (33 percent) (Maier, Hildebrandt, Klinger, Henrich-Eberl, & Lindena, 2002).

These findings paint a confusing picture of opioid therapy for chronic pain. In the end, the most commonly expressed view is that chronic opioid therapy can be used safely and effectively in carefully selected patients. Psychological evaluation is an essential component of patient selection for opioid treatment. Patient characteristics that raise concerns about chronic opioid therapy include psychopathology, a history of substance abuse or criminal activity, or personality disorders (Portenoy, 1996). Psychological evaluation is also paramount in ongoing assessment of responses to opioids. Regular assessment of pain, psychological function, and pain-related quality of life are imperative, and successful treatment should lead to improvements in each of these areas. Also, continued monitoring of compliance with medication regimens and aberrant drug behaviors is essential (Nedeljkovic, Wasan, & Jamison, 2002). Cognitive-behavioral therapy in conjunction with opioid treatment is also strongly recommended for most patients. Thus, a comprehensive, interdisciplinary approach to evaluation and treatment is needed in order to provide optimal management of chronic pain using long-term opioid therapy.

Oswestry Low Back Pain Disability Questionnaire: The Oswestry Low Back Pain Disability Questionnaire assesses the extent to which a person's function is impaired by back or leg pain (Fairbank, Couper, Davies, & O'Brien, 1980). It contains ten items, including a pain rating and nine items addressing the effect of pain on daily activities. A total score, the Oswestry Disability Index, is computed by summing the items and higher scores reflect greater disability. It is among the most widely used measures of disability in chronic pain populations, and substantial research supports its reliability and validity (Fairbank & Pynsent, 2000).

P

pain: Pain is defined as "an unpleasant sensory and emotional experience associated with actual or potential tissue damage or defined in terms of such damage" (Merskey & Bogduk, 1994, p. 210). It is important to recognize that pain is a personal experience rather than a set of neural events. Indeed, in expounding on the definition of pain, the Taxonomy Committee stated: "Activity induced in the nociceptor and nociceptive pathways by a noxious stimulus is not pain, which is always a psychological state" (Merskey & Bogduk, 1994, p. 210). One major feature of pain that distinguishes it from other sensations is its inherent unpleasantness. Because some other sensations are unpleasant but not painful (e.g., itch, some odors, and sounds), Fields (1999) recommended adding a new term, *algosity,* to our conceptualization of pain to connote the sensory aspect of an unpleasant sensory experience that allows us to recognize it as pain.

Some pain researchers have expressed concern regarding this definition of pain, due to its heavy emphasis on the subjective experience of pain and the reliance of verbal reports as the most valid pain measure (Anand & Craig, 1996). These authors discuss the difficulty of applying this definition to nonverbal organisms, including nonhuman animals, preverbal children, and individuals who are noncommunicative due to disability or cognitive impairment.

Distinctions among types of pain can be made based on the temporal characteristics of pain (i.e., acute versus chronic), or based on the known or suspected etiology of the pain, such as: inflammatory pain, neuropathic pain, musculoskeletal pain, visceral pain, or cancer pain. These distinctions are worth noting, as the quality of and psychological contributors to the pain may differ significantly across various types of pain.

pain assessment: Multiple methods for assessing pain are available, and they can be broadly classified as either self-report or not. In clinical settings, the most common method for assessing pain severity is an 11-point (i.e., from 0 to 10) numerical rating scale (NRS) (Jensen & Karoly, 2001). This method offers convenience for the assessor and ease of use for the patient, and NRSs appear relatively sensitive to treatment-related changes in pain. A criticism has been that NRSs do not actually provide ratio-level scaling of pain, which can be problematic more from a statistical than a practical point of view. Zero to 100 NRSs are also frequently used.

Another common method of pain assessment is verbal rating scales (VRS) in which the patient chooses a word that most accurately reflects his or her pain level (e.g., no pain, mild, moderate, severe). Although numbers are often assigned to each descriptor, VRS are actually categorical and not ordinal or ratio scales, unless numerical weights for the descriptors have been empirically determined and validated (e.g., Gracely, McGrath, & Dubner, 1978).

The visual analog scale (VAS) assesses pain by presenting patients with a line of predetermined length anchored at each end with descriptors (e.g., "no pain" and "most intense pain imaginable"). Patients place a mark bisecting the line to provide an estimate of their pain level, and the length of the line leading up to the mark is recorded. VASs have excellent statistical properties, including ratio-level scaling (Price, McGrath, Rafii, & Buckingham, 1983); however, they require more time to administer and score and some individuals have difficulty understanding the concept (Jensen & Karoly, 2001). Both mechanical and electronic VASs are available, which can enhance usability and reduce scoring errors.

In addition to these single-item pain measures, multiple-item pain measures are available, including the McGill Pain Questionnaire (MPQ), the Descriptor Differential Scale (DDS), and the Brief Pain Inventory (BPI), and these instruments provide more detailed assessment of pain. The DDS consists of two lists of 12 words, one for pain intensity and the other for pain affect, and patients rate the extent to which each word describes their pain level. This scale has excellent statistical properties but is somewhat cumbersome (Gracely & Kwilosz, 1988). Originally developed for assessment of pain in cancer patients, the BPI asks patients to rate their worst, least, average, and current pain levels using 11-point NRSs (Daut, Cleeland, & Flanery, 1983). Patients also rate the degree to which pain interferes in multiple aspects of life, and a pain drawing is included. This tool has been widely used with cancer patients; it provides information not only about pain severity but also pain-related interference and pain location. These scales have the disadvantage of requiring more time for administration and scoring, compared to single-item measures; however, they afford considerably more information. For example, the MPQ provides data regarding the quality of the pain, which can be helpful in determining diagnoses. Also, the BPI includes items related to the temporal characteristics and bodily location(s) of the pain. Thus, the increased time required for administration of these scales offers the advantage of more detailed information regarding the nature of the patient's pain.

Two types of pain-related measures do not rely on self-report, on observation of overt behavior, or physiological measures. Regarding behavioral measures, detailed systems for coding and quantifying overt pain behaviors exhibited by patients with clinical pain have been described and validated (Keefe, Fillingim, & Williams, 1991; Keefe, Wilkins, & Cook, 1984; Keefe et al., 1987; Keefe & Smith, 2002). Commonly observed pain behaviors include guarding (e.g., limping), rubbing the painful area, and facial grimacing. These behavioral measures have been correlated to patients' self-reported pain and depression. Pain behaviors increase in the presence of a solicitous spouse, and pain behaviors are reduced by multidisciplinary pain treatment (Keefe & Smith, 2002). A specific aspect of pain behavior that has received considerable attention is the analysis of facial expressions. Methods for classifying facial expressions have been well validated in emotion research (e.g., the Facial Action Coding System), and such systems have been successfully applied to experimental and clinical pain (Craig & Patrick, 1985; Craig, 1992). Behavioral observation methods are particularly useful when attempting to quantify pain in patients unable to provide verbal ratings (e.g., infants, cognitively impaired patients). Also, both in scientific and in clinical arenas, concerns are frequently expressed over the complete reliance on patients' self-reports of pain, and behavioral measures provides an additional source of data on which to base treatment decisions. Interestingly, pain behaviors and self-reported pain can provide conflicting information, which presents a dilemma for the clinician or scientist. It is important to remember that pain behavior, while more directly observable than self-report, is not necessarily a more valid or accurate measure of patients' pain.

Physiological measures of pain have long been sought, as clinicians and scientists desired more objective indices of pain. Autonomic responses were thought to be viable candidates, since noxious stimuli reliably elicit changes in measures such as blood pressure, heart rate, electrodermal responses, and pupil dilation. However, these responses are not specific to painful stimuli, as other emotional and physical stressors are able to evoke similar patterns of autonomic activation. Moreover, the experience of pain can be accompanied by increased responses on some autonomic indices but blunted responses on others, and substantial individual differences are present in physiological responses to painful stimulation. A variety of muscle reflexes (e.g., the nociceptive flexion reflex, exteroceptive suppression of the temporalis muscle) to noxious stimuli have been described, and these appear to be related to nociceptive processing. Indeed, such reflexes are correlated with pain report and are sensitive to analgesic treatments. However, due to the required expertise and resources for measuring such responses, these reflexes are primarily relegated to laboratory research. In addition, they represent neuromuscular responses to nociceptive stimuli and should be considered supplementary measures rather than a substitute for assessing the perceptual experience of pain.

In recent years, functional imaging has garnered tremendous attention in pain research. In humans, techniques such as single photon emission computed tomography (SPECT), positron emission tomography (PET), and functional magnetic resonance imaging (fMRI) have been applied to quantifying cerebral activity associated with clinical and/or experimentally induced pain. These imaging methods actually detect changes in regional cerebral blood flow (rCBF), which is closely related to synaptic activity. A discussion of the advantages and disadvantages of these various imaging methods is beyond the scope of this book, and readers are referred to Casey & Bushnell's (2000) recent book *Pain Imaging* for more detailed information. Imaging studies have revealed considerable, though not always consistent, information regarding pain-related cerebral responses. For example, some, but not all, clinical chronic pain conditions have been associated with decreased resting thalamic activation, and many clinical pain states are characterized by increased activity in the anterior cingulate cortex. These findings in clinical populations appear to vary depending on the nature of the pain (e.g., nociceptive versus neuropathic). Regarding experimentally induced pain, cutaneous pain generally produces activation in the thalamus, somatosensory cortices, and anterior cingulate and insular cortices (Rainville, 2002). The pattern of results appears to be influenced by the temporal attributes (e.g., phasic versus tonic), the location (e.g., cutaneous versus visceral), and the intensity of the painful stimuli. For example, pain-related activation in multiple brain regions became more robust and bilateral with increased stimulus intensity, suggesting good correspondence between cerebral and perceptual responses (Coghill, Sang, Maisog, & Iadarola, 1999). Brain imaging has also been used to examine endogenous pain modulation, and elegant studies using hypnotic suggestions have elucidated the neuroanatomical pathways involved in pain affect versus pain sensation (Rainville, Duncan, Price, Carrier, & Bushnell, 1997). Thus, pain imaging has yielded many important and valuable results.

Despite its successes, several limitations to these methods must be recognized. First, whether cerebral activation is "pain-related" is typically determined by measuring rCBF in certain regions of interest during pain stimulation and subtracting out rCBF in those same regions of interest that occurred during some control stimulation, typically an innocuous stimulus from the same modality. This approach assumes that the only difference between the painful and control-stimulation conditions is pain; however, this is rarely the case. For example, painful stimulation is typically more attentionally demanding, more anxiety provoking, and may involve greater cortical effort devoted to suppressing motor responses. It may be these components of the pain condition, rather than the pain itself, that produce increased activation in some brain regions. In addition, increased rCBF, which reflects increased synaptic activity, could indicate either excitatory or inhibitory neural responses. In the latter case, one would expect increased activation to be related to decreased intensity of pain. Finally, these technologies remain quite expensive, require highly specialized equipment and facilities, and demand considerable expertise; therefore, their integration into routine clinical assessment is not imminent. Nonetheless, pain imaging represents a promising approach for translational pain research and will undoubtedly expedite understanding of the neural transmission of pain in humans.

pain threshold and tolerance: *Pain threshold* refers to "the least experience of pain which a subject can recognize" (Merskey & Bogduk, 1994, p. 213). Numerous methods are available for determining pain threshold, and the actual value of pain threshold is dependent on the subjective criteria used to consider a sensation painful (Gracely, 1994). *Pain tolerance* is defined as "the greatest level of pain which a subject is prepared to tolerate" (Merskey & Bogduk, 1994, p. 213). As with pain threshold, pain tolerance can be determined via numerous methods and is thought to be more dependent on motivational factors. Substantial research indicates that both pain threshold and tolerance are significantly influenced by numerous psychological factors, including mood, coping, and motivation (see Gracely, 1994, for a review).

palliative care: Palliative care refers to treatment directed at symptom management and enhanced quality of life, typically in the context of progressive or terminal illness. Pain is highly prevalent among patients with cancer and AIDS, and unique psychosocial aspects of pain may occur in these populations (Breitbart & Payne, 2004). In patients with cancer or AIDS, pain is associated with increased suffering, poorer quality of life, and suicidal ideation and those patients who interpret pain as a sign of disease progression show more pain-related distress and disability than those who attribute pain to benign causes (Breitbart & Payne, 2004). As with other forms of pain, cognitive-behavioral interventions are effective for reducing pain and emotional distress among patients with progressive medical illnesses (Devine, 2003). Among patients with terminal illness, the primary goal of psychological therapy often becomes support for both the patient and family. Thus, psychological factors and treatments are very important in providing optimal palliative care.

patient-centered treatment: The patient-centered model of health care delivery emphasizes that the patient's views should be recognized and appreciated. This model incorporates the patient's perspective into treatment decisions and outcome evaluation, and has been adopted as a goal of clinical medicine (Laine & Davidoff, 1996). Use of this model can produce greater satisfaction with health care, improved compliance with medical regimens, and enhancement of patient-provider relationships (Fischer et al., 1999). This model is highly relevant to the treatment of chronic pain, but little research has been conducted in this area. One important issue in patient-centered care is the determination of patients' desired treatment outcomes. In this regard, Casarett, Karlawish, Sankar, Hirschman, & Asch (2001) interviewed patients with chronic pain relevant to the clinical improvements that they hoped for from a new medication. The average patient identified five clinical endpoints that a new medication could address in order to represent an improvement over current therapy. The most frequent choices were: decreased pain, increased activities of daily living, improved sleep, and improved mood. Relatedly, patients' ratings of their criteria for judging treatment as successful and the importance of improvement across multiple symptom domains (i.e., pain, interference, fatigue, mood) were assessed in 52 patients with back pain (Robinson et al., in press). Patients rated improvements across all four domains as important to them and their success criteria required greater than 50 percent deductions across all domains. Thus, patients are desirous of substantial improvements along multiple symptom dimensions, not just pain.

One important component of the patient-centered approach is tailoring treatment to the patient's needs. Although this has been recommended in pain treatment (*see* MULTIDIMENSIONAL PAIN INVENTORY), limited implementation of treatment tailoring has occurred. One recent study examined the effectiveness of training physicians in a communication-based patient-centered approach for treating patients with musculoskeletal pain (Alamo, Moral, & Perula de Torres, 2002). Compared to the standard care group, patients who received the patient-centered approach showed greater improvements in anxiety and number of tender points, and trends showed improvement in clinical pain. Undoubtedly, the patient-centered model will be increasingly applied to pain assessment and treatment in the future.

pelvic pain: Chronic pelvic pain (CPP) refers to a cluster of visceral pain syndromes affecting the pelvic region. Pelvic pain predominantly affects women, though not exclusively, as chronic prostatitis is a common pain syndrome in men (McNaughton, 2003; Stones & Price, 2002; Zondervan & Barlow, 2000; Schaeffer, 2003). Estimates of the prevalence of CPP in women range from 14.7 to 24 percent, with the majority of sufferers not seeking health care for their condition (Stones, Selfe, Fransman, & Horn, 2000; Zondervan & Barlow, 2000). Nonetheless, CPP is a frequent primary complaint prompting visits to a gynecologist, and a large number of laparoscopies and hysterectomies are performed to treat CPP (Stones et al., 2000; Zondervan & Barlow, 2000). CPP can result from numerous underlying conditions, including pelvic inflammatory disease, pelvic congestion syndrome, endometriosis, interstitial cystitits, musculoskeletal pain, and gastrointestinal conditions (Moore & Kennedy, 2000). Among men, chronic prostatitis/prostatodynia is the most common pelvic pain condition. The etiology is poorly understood, though prostatitis-like symptoms can be due to dysfunction of pelvic floor muscles or myofascial pain, and treatment outcomes are generally unimpressive (McNaughton, 2003; Wesselmann, Burnett, & Heinberg, 1997; Schaeffer, 2003; Potts, 2003).

Psychological factors are believed important among both women and men experiencing CPP. For example, a self-reported history of sexual abuse is more common among women with CPP (Heim, Ehlert, Hanker, & Hellhammer, 1998; Reed et al., 2000; Toomey, Hernandez, Gittelman, & Hulka, 1993), though this finding has been reported for many other pain syndromes as well (*see* ABUSE). Women with CPP also report a greater number of stressful life events, and some investigators have reported higher levels of depression among women with CPP compared to healthy controls (McNaughton, 2003; Reed et al., 2000; Bodden-Heidrich et al., 1999; Heim et al., 1998; Waller & Shaw, 1995). Given the association of psychological disturbance with CPP, a multidisciplinary approach to treatment, including psychological treatment along with medical/surgical intervention, has been recommended (Stones & Price, 2002; Wesselmann et al.,

1997; Milburn, Reiter, & Rhomberg, 1993). The limited available evidence suggests that this approach may be beneficial (Stones & Mountfield, 2000; Milburn et al., 1993), and more controlled trials are needed to determine the effectiveness of psychological therapies in this patient population.

personality: Personality refers to *enduring* psychological characteristics and features that influence an individual's thoughts, feelings, and behaviors. Personality characteristics are generally established by early adulthood, and genetics make a substantial contribution to personality (Bouchard Jr. & McGue, 2003; Eid, Riemann, Angleitner, & Borkenau, 2003; Jang, Livesley, & Vernon, 1996). Numerous theories of personality are available, including psychodynamic theories, trait theories, humanistic theories, and behavioral theories. Two major lines of investigation supporting the influence of personality on chronic pain are: (1) studies involving personality assessment among patients with chronic pain, and (2) studies of personality disorders in chronic pain populations.

Regarding the assessment of personality characteristics, numerous studies demonstrated higher levels of personality dysfunction among patients with chronic pain compared to pain-free controls. For example, higher levels of neuroticism have been reported (*see* NEUROTICISM), and elevations on multiple MMPI scales are characteristic (*see* MINNESOTA MULTIPHASIC PERSONALITY INVENTORY). Thus, maladaptive personality profiles are common among chronic pain populations. In addition, considerable data indicate that personality disorders are more common in chronic pain populations. Personality disorders are psychiatric diagnoses that emerge when personality traits are inflexible, maladaptive, and cause significant impairment or subjective distress (American Psychiatric Association, 1994). Several studies using structured interviews have documented increased prevalence of personality disorders among patients with chronic pain than in the general population (Weisberg & Keefe, 1999). Thus, personality factors represent important variables to consider in the assessment and management of persons with chronic pain.

phantom limb pain: Phantom limb pain (PLP) is the experience of pain in a limb that has been amputated, and this occurs in 50 to 80 percent of amputees (Jensen, Krebs, Nielsen, & Rasmussen, 1985; Katz

& Gagliese, 1999). Phantom limb pain occurs in children and adults, but the experience of PLP appears to be rare in individuals with a congenitally missing limb (Flor, 2002; Katz & Gagliese, 1999). PLP was more common in lower than in upper limbs in one recent study (Dijkstra, Geertzen, Stewart, & van der Schans, 2002). Historically, psychological explanations, especially psychodynamic ones, were offered to explain the presence of PLP. However, while quality of life is poorer in amputees with phantom pain compared to amputees without pain, no convincing evidence has been found that psychological factors are instrumental in the etiology of PLP, as carefully conducted studies demonstrate few psychological differences between amputees with versus without PLP (see Katz & Gagliese, 1999, for a review). The most compelling explanation for PLP is that following deafferentation reorganization occurs at multiple levels of the central nervous system, including the somatosensory and motor cortices, the thalamus, the brainstem, and perhaps the spinal cord (Flor, 2002).

Although they are not etiologic, psychological factors do contribute to pain-related adjustment among patients with PLP (Sherman, Sherman, & Bruno, 1987). For example, pain coping predicts the intensity of pain as well as the amount of pain-related psychological and physical dysfunction (Hill, Niven, & Knussen, 1995). Also, Jensen and colleagues (2002) recently examined several psychological factors as predictors of pain intensity, pain-related interference, and depression among patients with PLP. Catastrophizing and the use of pain-contingent rest as a coping strategy predicted higher pain levels and increased pain-related interference. Higher levels of social support predicted greater reductions in pain over a five-month period, while higher levels of solicitous responding by significant others predicted less pain improvement. These findings indicate the important role of psychological factors in adjustment to PLP and suggest that incorporating psychological treatment into the management of PLP will enhance outcomes.

placebo: Although a placebo is often conceptualized as a treatment designed to mimic an actual therapy but without active ingredients, the placebo response is a therapeutic effect of a treatment that is not due to the active ingredient(s) of that treatment. This distinction is especially important for analgesic interventions, as placebo analgesia is a well-documented phenomenon. Several factors contribute to the magnitude of placebo analgesia, the most important of which is patients' expectations of pain relief; however, patients' desire for pain relief and the role of conditioning (i.e., previous exposure to an effective analgesic intervention) are also important (Benedetti, Arduino, & Amanzio, 1999; Price et al., 1999). The placebo phenomenon should be recognized as a component of the response to any intervention. For example, following thoracotomy, patients were administered saline placebo under one of three instructional conditions: (1) hidden injection with no instruction, (2) instruction that the injection could be a painkiller or a placebo (double-blind), and (3) instruction that they were receiving a powerful painkiller (deceptive placebo) (Pollo et al., 2001). The three groups of patients were then observed over three days, and their pain levels and postoperative consumption of the opioid buprenorphine were recorded. Postoperative pain was similar across the three conditions; however, patients in the deceptive placebo group consumed 34 percent less buprenorphine than the hidden injection group and 16 percent less than the double-blind instruction group. Thus, the placebo instruction significantly increased the effectiveness of buprenorphine in this group. Substantial evidence now indicates that placebo analgesia is mediated at least in part by activation of endogenous opioids, since naloxone, an opioid receptor antagonist, can reverse placebo responses (Benedetti et al., 1999; Benedetti & Amanzio, 1997; Levine, Gordon, & Fields, 1978). From a psychological perspective, placebo analgesia represents an impressive demonstration that cognitive variables can alter pain via direct neurobiological effects on nociceptive processing.

postoperative pain: The management of postoperative pain is a significant issue. There were 31.5 million outpatient surgeries in 1996 and 40 million inpatient surgeries in 2001 (National Center for Health Statistics, 2004). Patients expect pain following surgery, but the evidence suggests that postoperative pain continues to be poorly controlled, with large proportions of patients experiencing moderate to severe pain (Apfelbaum, Chen, Mehta, & Gan, 2003; Huang, Cunningham, Laurito, & Chen, 2001; Strassels, Chen, & Carr, 2002). Interestingly, patients report being generally satisfied with postoperative pain management, even though they experience moderate to severe pain (Strassels et al., 2002). However, patient satisfaction is not the only endpoint to consider. Improved pain control following surgery can reduce costs and improve medical outcomes (Kehlet & Dahl, 2003; Kehlet & Holte, 2001; Strassels et al., 2002).

Numerous studies demonstrate the contribution of psychological factors to postoperative pain. For example, preoperative anxiety is a significant predictor of postoperative pain and analgesic consumption (Caumo et al., 2002; Gil, Ginsberg, Muir, Sykes, & Williams, 1990; Nelson, Zimmerman, Barnason, Nieveen, & Schmaderer, 1998; Perry, Parker, White, & Clifford, 1994). Moreover, psychological interventions can reduce postoperative pain. For instance, the use of imagery, in which patients imagined coping effectively with postoperative symptoms, reduced postoperative pain and analgesic use among patients undergoing colorectal surgery (Manyande et al., 1995). Similarly, the use of relaxation, music, or the combination was associated with lower pain following gynecologic surgery compared to no treatment (Good, Anderson, Stanton-Hicks, Grass, & Makii, 2002). Also, hypnosis has been shown to significantly reduce postoperative pain and anxiety compared to an active control condition (Faymonville et al., 1997), and some preliminary evidence suggests that hypnosis may improve surgical wound healing (Ginandes, Brooks, Sando, Jones, & Aker, 2003). These data suggest that postoperative pain remains a significant clinical problem which is influenced by psychological factors, and psychological interventions can be effective in reducing pain after surgery.

post-traumatic stress disorder: Post-traumatic stress disorder (PTSD) is a psychiatric disorder characterized by the development of anxiety-related symptoms following exposure to a traumatic event (American Psychiatric Association, 1994). Symptoms of PTSD include: persistently reexperiencing the event (e.g., intrusive memories, nightmares), avoidance of associated stimuli, and symptoms of increased arousal (e.g., hypervigilance, difficulty sleeping). Because chronic pain often results from traumatic injury (e.g., motor vehicle accidents, work-related injuries), it seems feasible that PTSD and chronic pain may occur at the same time. Indeed, PTSD is more frequent among chronic pain patients than in the general population (McWilliams, Cox, & Enns, 2003), and among individuals who have suffered a traumatic brain injury, those with chronic pain were more likely to report PTSD than those without chronic pain (Bryant, Marosszeky, Crooks, Baguley, & Gurka, 1999). Recent review articles discussed several factors that may contribute to a mutual maintenance between chronic pain and PTSD, including: attentional biases, anxiety sensitivity, avoidant coping, depression, and heightened pain sensitivity (Sharp & Harvey, 2001; Asmundson, Coons, Taylor, & Katz, 2002). Moreover, alterations in hypothalamic-pituitary-adrenal (HPA) axis function have been associated with both PTSD and chronic pain and may represent an additional mechanism whereby these conditions are linked (Ehlert, Gaab, & Heinrichs, 2001). Additional research is needed to elucidate the reasons for the overlap between chronic pain and PTSD and to inform treatment of these comorbid conditions.

prayer: In recent years, the role of spirituality and religiosity in health has garnered increased attention. In general medical patients, religious coping has been associated with lower levels of depression and less physical disability (Koenig, 2002). For chronic pain, however, prayer typically has been conceptualized as a passive and maladaptive coping strategy, and most studies have shown that patients who report frequent use of prayer also report higher levels of pain (Keefe & Dolan, 1986; Rosenstiel & Keefe, 1983). Interestingly, one study found that over time, increased use of praying and hoping was associated with decreased pain (Turner & Clancy, 1986). A recent study identified both positive and negative components of religious coping among patients with chronic pain (Bush et al., 1999). Positive religious coping involves drawing strength and comfort from God, while negative religious coping includes appraisals that one is being punished or has been abandoned by God. However, in the sample studied, these religious coping variables were not predictive of pain-related adjustment. Nonetheless, recognizing the multidimensionality of religious coping will be important in future research on this topic. Koenig (2002) discusses several mechanisms whereby religious coping, including prayer, can improve health conditions. These include giving patients an enhanced sense of control, reducing feelings of helplessness, promoting relaxation, providing social support (e.g., through church attendance), and serving as a distraction. Moreover, religious coping often occurs in the context of an optimistic worldview that leads the patient to engage in more constructive appraisals of his or her medical condition. Thus, religious coping/ prayer may represent adaptive strategies for coping with chronic pain, but additional research is needed to understand whether and how this approach influences pain-related adjustment.

psychodynamic theory: Psychodynamic theory dominated thinking about psychological functioning for the first half of the twentieth century, and it remains an influential theory to this day. The primary tenet of psychodynamic theory is that our personality is shaped by our efforts to reduce conflict or to balance the energy of different forces within our minds. Psychodynamic theory also proposed that many of our thoughts and feelings remain hidden from our awareness, in our unconscious. Freud's well-known theory proposed that intrapsychic conflict arising from our sexual and aggressive impulses was central, and other psychodynamic theorists focused on other sources of conflict. According to Freudian theory, conversion represents one mechanism whereby psychic conflict could be reduced (*see* CONVERSION DISORDER). More recent formulations emphasize relational aspects of psychodynamic theory, such that our patterns of relating to others shape our personalities (Basler, Grzesiak, & Dworkin, 2002). Though many therapists have abandoned psychodynamic theories for the more tangible cognitive-behavioral approaches, psychodynamic concepts continue to influence the conceptualization and treatment of patients. Thus, it is important to recognize and integrate these concepts into the understanding of chronic pain.

psychogenic pain: In the era of psychodynamic theory, pain that could not readily be explained based on documented medical findings was often deemed *psychogenic* (i.e., caused by psychic conflict). In a classic paper titled "Psychogenic Pain and the Pain-Prone Patient," Engel (1959) described several characteristics of pain whereby it takes on a "central position in psychic development and function" (p. 901). Pain (1) warns of potential bodily damage; (2) is intricately involved in human relationships; (3) is linked with punishment starting early in development; (4) becomes associated with aggression and power early in childhood; (5) becomes associated with actual or imagined loss of loved ones; and (6) may be associated with sexual feelings. Based on these potential meanings of pain, he noted three conditions under which psychogenic pain is likely to occur: (1) when external circumstances fail to satisfy the unconscious need to suffer;

(2) as a response to real, imagined, or fantasied loss; or (3) when guilt is evoked by intense aggressive or forbidden sexual feelings.

Purely psychogenic pain appears to be a rare occurrence and psychogenic pain is no longer a psychiatric diagnosis. The replacement diagnosis in the DSM-IV is *pain disorder,* which refers to a condition in which pain is the predominant clinical focus, pain causes impairment or distress, and psychological factors are thought to have an important role in the onset, severity, exacerbation, or maintenance of the pain (American Psychiatric Association, 1994). It seems appropriate to avoid the term *psychogenic,* as the prevalence of pain that is truly caused by psychological factors seems to be exceedingly low. Moreover, the term evokes dualistic conceptualizations of pain, in which biological and psychological contributions were mutually exclusive.

psychophysics: Psychophysics has been defined as the scientific study of the relation between stimulus and sensation, and it played a major role in the development of experimental psychology (Gescheider, 1997). When specifically applied to pain, psychophysical methods are used to quantify the perception of painful stimuli. The most common methods in pain psychophysics involve assessment of pain threshold (*see* PAIN THRESHOLD AND TOLERANCE); however, numerous additional methods exist. To discuss psychophysics, one must consider both stimulus and sensation. Regarding the former, multiple experimental pain stimuli are available, including mechanical, thermal, electrical, ischemic, and chemical stimuli (for detailed reviews see Curatolo, Petersen-Felix, & Arendt-Nielsen, 2000; Gracely, 1994). These stimuli differ along several important dimensions, including temporal characteristics, depth of tissue stimulated, selectivity of afferent fibers stimulated, and the clinical relevance of the pain experienced. In order to assess sensation (i.e., pain perception), the methods described in the "pain assessment" section are typically used.

Pain psychophysics can serve several important purposes (for a more detailed discussion see Fillingim & Lautenbacher, 2003): Pain psychophysics

- has been widely used to examine dispositional and situational factors that influence pain perception
- can be extremely helpful for investigating the mechanisms underlying normal and abnormal pain perception

- can be used to enhance diagnosis of patients with pain disorders
- can be used to improve the assessment of clinical pain severity
- can be an effective outcome measure for documenting treatment responses in patients undergoing various interventions

The clinical use of pain psychophysics, or quantitative sensory testing, has increased significantly in recent years, and researchers hope that this type of testing will enhance pain diagnosis and treatment.

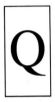

quality of life: Quality of life is a vague term that refers to patients' perceived well-being in several areas of functioning, including psychological, physical, social, and spiritual. In biomedical research, health-related quality of life has become a frequently used measure of the impact of chronic illness on an individual's overall well-being. The terms health-related quality of life (HRQOL) and general health status are often used interchangeably, and several instruments commonly used to assess HRQOL are available (McDowell & Newell, 1996).

One of the most commonly used measures is the Short Form 36 Health Survey (SF-36), developed by the Rand Corporation for survey research on health status, including the Medical Outcomes Study (MOS) (Ware Jr. & Sherbourne, 1992). The SF-36 includes 36 items drawn form the original 245-item MOS questionnaire, and it measures the following eight dimensions of health status:

1. physical functioning,
2. role limitations due to physical health problems,
3. bodily pain,
4. social functioning,
5. general mental health,
6. role limitations due to emotional problems,
7. vitality, energy, or fatigue, and
8. general health perceptions.

The SF-36 has good psychometric properties and has been used extensively to assess health status in multiple chronic medical conditions (McHorney, Ware Jr., Lu, & Sherbourne, 1994; McHorney, Ware Jr., & Raczek, 1993). The SF-36 has been used in numerous chronic pain populations, including headache, chronic back pain, irritable bowel syndrome, arthritis, and fibromyalgia, and the results demonstrate significantly diminished quality of life in each of these conditions (Fanciullo et al., 2003; Daffner et al., 2003; Harpole et al., 2003; Guitera, Munoz, Castillo, & Pascual, 2002; Gralnek, Hays, Kilbourne, Naliboff, & Mayer, 2000). The SF-36 has also been sensitive to treatment outcome in chronic pain populations (Harpole et al., 2003; Ruoff, Rosenthal, Jordan, Karim, & Kamin, 2003).

Another commonly used HRQOL measure, the Sickness Impact Profile (SIP), assesses the impact of sickness on daily activities and behaviors (Bergner, Bobbitt, Carter, & Gilson, 1981; Bergner, Bobbitt, Pollard, Martin, & Gilson, 1976). The final version includes 136 items describing specific behavior changes (e.g., "I am not working at all," "I walk shorter distances or stop to rest often") across 12 categories, including physical and psychosocial dimensions. A strength of the SIP is its reliance on behavioral end points rather than global perceptions or feelings. A potential disadvantage is its length, though shortened versions have been validated (de Bruin, Buys, de Witte, & Diederiks, 1994; de Bruin, Diederiks, de Witte, Stevens, & Philipsen, 1994). The SIP has been used to assess general health status in myriad medical populations, including patients with arthritis, fibromyalgia, low back pain, abdominal pain, and heterogeneous chronic pain samples (de Bruin, de Witte, Stevens, & Diederiks, 1992; Jensen, Strom, Turner, & Romano, 1992; Watt-Watson & Graydon, 1989; Follick, Smith, & Ahern, 1985; Martin et al., 1996).

A number of additional generic and disease-specific HRQOL measures are available but will not be reviewed here. The interested reader is referred elsewhere for more detailed information on available instruments for assessing HRQOL (McDowell & Newell, 1996). Measures of health-related quality of life/general health status should be integrated into chronic pain assessment, as these are important indicators of the impact of chronic pain as well as the overall benefits of treatment.

R

reflex sympathetic dystrophy: *See* COMPLEX REGIONAL PAIN SYNDROME.

relaxation training: Relaxation training is one of the cornerstones of cognitive-behavioral coping skills training for chronic pain. Multiple methods of relaxation training are available, including progressive muscle relaxation, autogenic training, and guided imagery. Relaxation training can be conducted with or without biofeedback assistance (*see* BIOFEEDBACK). As with biofeedback and cognitive-behavioral treatment, numerous controlled trials demonstrate that relaxation treatment is effective for reducing both acute and chronic pain (Spence, Sharpe, Newton-John, & Champion, 1995; Rokicki et al., 1997; ter Kuile et al., 1994; Luebbert, Dahme, & Hasenbring, 2001; Holroyd & Penzien, 1990; Arena & Blanchard, 1996; Eccleston, Yorke, Morley, Williams, & Mastroyannopoulou, 2003). Relaxation therapy is easily integrated into pain management and the vast majority of patients are capable of learning relaxation techniques. Thus, relaxation represents an efficacious nonpharmacological therapy that readily can be integrated into a patient's pain management regimen.

reliability: Reliability of an assessment method refers to that method's ability to provide consistent measurement. Common forms of reliability include test-retest reliability, which reflects consistency of measurement over time, and inter-rater reliability, which reflects consistency of measurement across different raters. Another important aspect of reliability is internal consistency, which indicates whether individual items on a measure assess the same construct. The contribution of error to variability in pain responses increases as the reliability of the pain measure decreases. Thus, unreliable measures are less capable of detecting actual changes in pain that may occur between individuals or over time. It is also important to realize that reliability sets the ceiling on validity (*see* VALIDITY), such that an unreliable measure cannot be valid. When evaluating pain research, it is important to consider the reliability (and validity) of the measures used. The importance of understanding reliability and validity and further information on these concepts is provided in a recent article by Jensen (2003).

religion/spirituality: *See* PRAYER.

secondary gain: As discussed previously (*see* CONVERSION DISORDER), secondary gain refers to external benefits that patients may receive contingent on their pain and pain-related behavior. Secondary gain is also known as reinforcement in behavioral parlance (*see* BEHAVIORAL FACTORS), and the net effect of secondary gain is to increase the frequency of pain behavior. Common secondary gain factors that clinicians attend to are disability payments, pending litigation, overly solicitous spouses, and avoidance of aversive tasks or situations. The roles of these factors have been discussed in more detail in previous sections. (*See* BEHAVIORAL FACTORS; FAMILY; LEGAL ISSUES.)

self-efficacy: Self-efficacy refers to the belief that one can accomplish an outcome through one's own efforts. The concept of self-efficacy was developed by Albert Bandura in the context of his social cognitive theory (Bandura, 1997). The concept of self-efficacy is important for pain research. For example, individuals' beliefs in their ability to tolerate pain (i.e., their self-efficacy for pain tolerance) predict their actual pain responses in laboratory settings (Baker & Kirsch, 1991; Bandura, O'Leary, Taylor, Gauthier, & Gossard, 1987; Dolce et al., 1986; Lowery, Fillingim, & Wright, 2003). Also, college students who reported persistent pain had lower self-efficacy ratings compared to pain-free individuals (Karoly & Lecci, 1997). Pain-related self-efficacy is an important predictor of pain-related adjustment in patients with chronic pain. For example, in patients with low back pain and patients with cancer pain, perceived self-efficacy was inversely correlated with pain interference and severity (Lin, 1998). Also, after controlling for pain severity, patients' self-efficacy for pain control was inversely associated with psychological distress, and self-efficacy predicted activity levels in patients with low to moderate pain severity (Jensen & Karoly, 1991). In a study of low back pain patients, perceived functional self-efficacy predicted lifting performance (Lackner & Carosella, 1999), and functional self-efficacy predicted pain-related disability among veterans with chronic pain, even after controlling for pain intensity, number of pain sites, depression and other chronic conditions (Barry, Guo, Kerns, Duong, & Reid, 2003). In addition, numerous studies demonstrate an association between self-efficacy and arthritis-related pain and disability (Strahl, Kleinknecht, & Dinnel, 2000; Keefe et al., 2002; Marks, 2001). Self-efficacy also mediates the relationship between pain intensity and disability among patients with chronic pain (Arnstein, 2000; Arnstein, Caudill, Mandle, Norris, & Beasley, 1999).

Self-efficacy is an important predictor of progression of pain-related symptoms. In patients with knee osteoarthritis (OA), self-efficacy interacted with knee strength to predict declines in self-reported disability and functional performance over a 30-month period, such that patients with low self-efficacy and low strength showed the greatest reductions in these measures over time (Rejeski, Miller, Foy, Messier, & Rapp, 2001). In another study of knee OA, high levels of self-efficacy were associated with better functional outcomes over a three-year period (Sharma et al., 2003). Among patients with chronic low back pain, pain self-efficacy beliefs were negatively correlated with total pain behavior and avoidant behavior over a nine-month follow-up period. Taken together, these findings suggest that self-efficacy protects against functional declines and increases in pain behavior that may occur over time among patients with chronic pain.

Self-efficacy may also mediate treatment outcomes. Several studies demonstrate that nonpharmacological treatment for chronic pain produces increases in self-efficacy. For example, a supervised fitness program added to education produced significant increases in self-efficacy among patients with chronic low back pain compared to patients who attended only the educational program (Frost, Klaber Moffett, Moser, & Fairbank, 1995). Similarly, several years of outcome studies examining the Arthritis Self-Management Program (ASMP) reveal that this intervention results in significant improvement in self-efficacy (Lorig & Holman, 2003). A modification of the ASMP for patients with other forms of chronic pain has also demonstrated that self-efficacy increases with treatment (Frost et al., 1995). Moreover, these changes have been found to predict treatment-associated improvements in pain-related adjustment. Indeed, Lorig and colleagues reported that both baseline self-efficacy and changes in self-efficacy during treatment are positive predictors of treatment outcome from ASMP (Lorig & Holman, 2003; Lorig, Gonzalez, & Ritter, 1999). Other investigators observed an association between treatment-related increases in self-efficacy and clinical improvements following psychological intervention in patients with arthritis (Keefe et al., 1996, 1999; Smarr et al., 1997). Similar findings were reported for heterogeneous samples of chronic pain patients undergoing multidisciplinary rehabilitation (Jensen, Turner, & Romano, 1994, 2001).

These findings suggest that enhancing self-efficacy should be an important goal of pain treatment. Bandura (1997) proposes that self-efficacy can be altered in several ways. First, it can be increased by enacting a behavior; therefore, treatment programs that involve having patients perform activities in which they may otherwise not engage will be particularly helpful (e.g., exercise, active rehearsal of coping strategies). Second, self-efficacy can be enhanced through vicarious experience, such that group treatment, which affords opportunities for patients to observe successful coping attempts by others, may be beneficial. Third, it can be improved through verbal persuasion, which can come in the form of encouragement and education not only from providers, but also from other patients and family members. Fourth, self-efficacy can be reduced by the presence of physiological arousal states, such as those accompanying anxiety or fear. Thus, interventions that reduce anxiety and physiological arousal (e.g., relaxation, cognitive therapy) may enhance self-efficacy. This brief discussion indicates that many nonpharmacologic forms of pain treatment provide important conditions for enhancing self-efficacy.

serotonin: Serotonin, or 5-hydroxytryptamine (5-HT), is a neurotransmitter involved in numerous functions, including pain modulation, mood control, and sleep regulation. Direct influences of serotonergic systems on pain can be through actions at peripheral sites (e.g., in the gut) or through descending modulation of central nociceptive transmission. In addition, serotonin can influence pain responses indirectly, through effects on mood, sleep, or other functions that affect pain.

The peripheral actions of serotonin are considered to be pronociceptive. For example, total blood serotonin levels were negatively correlated with pressure pain threshold in healthy individuals (Pickering, Januel, Dubray, & Eschalier, 2003), and serum serotonin was positively correlated with tender-point count in patients with fibromyalgia (Wolfe, Russell, Vipraio, Ross, & Anderson, 1997). Moreover, serotonin levels in both serum and synovial fluid were positively correlated with pain severity in rheumatoid arthritis involving the temporomandibular joint (Kopp & Alstergren, 2002; Alstergren & Kopp, 1997). In addition, injection of serotonin into the masseter muscle produced spontaneous pain and significantly reduced the pressure-pain threshold in healthy females (Ernberg, Lundeberg, & Kopp, 2000b), and coinjection of granisetron, a 5-HT3 receptor antagonist, reduced the spontaneous pain and completely reversed the hyperalgesia (Ernberg, Lundeberg, & Kopp, 2000a).

Peripheral actions of serotonin are also relevant to irritable bowel syndrome, as both excitatory and inhibitory 5-HT receptors are in the gastrointestinal tract, and activation of these receptors can alter sensory and motor functions in the gut (Hansen, 2003). Because agonists and antagonists for different receptor subtypes can produce effects on both sensory (i.e., pain) and motor (i.e., gastrointestinal motility) responses, their clinical effects can be quite complex. Moreover, these drugs can also alter nociceptive processing via central nervous system effects. Although clinical efficacy in IBS has been demonstrated for agonists and antagonists at specific receptor 5-HT subtypes, adverse effects continue to be a concern (Talley, 2003; Hansen, 2003).

Serotonergic activity is also implicated in migraine headache, as agonists at the 5-HT_1 receptor (i.e., triptans) are effective antimigraine therapies (Durham & Russo, 2002). These medications are thought to work by both peripheral actions, including vasoconstriction of meningeal and cerebral blood vessels and inhibiting release of excitatory neuropeptides from trigeminal nerves, as well as by central effects (i.e., inhibition of trigeminal brain stem projection neurons) (Durham & Russo, 2002). Thus, peripheral and central effects of serotonergic drugs likely contribute to the benefits of serotonergic drugs for treatment of IBS and migraine.

Central serotonergic neurons also play a general role in pain responses primarily via descending pain modulation. Serotonergic neurons originating in the rostroventral medulla and the nucleus raphe magnus project to the spinal dorsal horn and the trigeminal brainstem, where they act upon nociceptive projection neurons (Millan, 2002). Classically, descending serotonergic neurons are considered as predominantly inhibitory; however, ample evidence indicates excitatory effects as well, which is due to the presence of multiple receptor subtypes and effects on different target neurons (e.g., primary afferents, interneurons, and projection neurons) (Millan, 2002). Clinical evidence suggests a central serotonergic dysfunction in fibromyalgia. For instance, lower levels of serum serotonin and its precursor, tryptophan, were reported in patients with fibromyalgia, which are believed to reflect lower central serotonergic activity (Russell, Michalek, Vipraio, Fletcher, & Wall, 1989; Wolfe et al., 1997; Yunus, Dailey, Aldag, Masi, & Jobe, 1992). Indeed, low levels of the serotonin metabolite, 5-HIAA, have been reported in the cerebrospinal fluid (CSF) of patients with fibromyalgia, providing more direct evidence of diminished central serotonergic function in this patient population (Legangneux et al., 2001). Thus, the direct effects of serotonergic systems on pain responses are complex and occur at all levels of the nociceptive processing system.

Serotonin also produces indirect effects on pain though its influence on sleep and mood, which may in turn alter pain responses. Indeed, sleep and mood disturbance are characteristic of chronic pain, and both sleep and mood disturbance can exacerbate pain. Therefore, dysregulation of the serotonin system that results in sleep and mood disturbance can amplify pain, and pharmacologic therapy that ameliorates sleep and mood problems via serotonergic mechanisms (e.g., antidepressant therapy) can attenuate pain.

sexual abuse: *See* ABUSE.

sleep disorders: The vast majority of patients with chronic pain report sleep disturbances, especially difficulties initiating and maintaining sleep. A high frequency of sleep disturbance was reported for patients with fibromyalgia, headache, orofacial pain, pelvic pain, and for heterogeneous samples of patients with chronic pain (Harding, 1998; Moldofsky, 1989; Sayar, Arikan, & Yontem, 2002; McCracken & Iverson, 2002; Riley III et al., 2001; Morin, Gibson, & Wade, 1998; Wilson, Watson, & Currie, 1998; Spierings & van Hoof, 1997; Haythornthwaite, Hegel, & Kerns, 1991; Pilowsky, Crettenden, & Townley, 1985). Moreover, in the general population, pain is a predictor of insomnia (Sutton, Moldofsky, & Badley, 2001; Henderson et al., 1995). Although most investigators have relied on self-report measures of sleep impairment, sleep studies involving electroencephalographic (EEG) assessments of sleep architecture also demonstrated significant sleep abnormalities associated with chronic pain (Schneider-Helmert, Whitehouse, Kumar, & Lijzenga, 2001; Dunlap, Yu, Fisch, & Nolan, 1998; Wittig, Zorick, Blumer, Heilbronn, & Roth, 1982). Among patients with chronic pain, sleep disruption is associated with more severe pain, pain of longer duration, greater disability, and increased emotional distress (Sayar et al., 2002; McCracken & Iverson, 2002; Riley III et al., 2001; Morin et al., 1998; Wilson et al., 1998; Haythornthwaite et al., 1991; Pilowsky et al., 1985).

Several mechanisms could explain the association between pain and sleep disturbance. First, chronic pain may cause sleep disturbance, as the presence of pain would be expected to disrupt sleep. Indeed, several investigations in healthy subjects suggest that the application of painful stimuli during sleep produce arousal in the EEG signal, though typically not causing the subject to awaken (Bentley, Newton, & Zio, 2003; Foo & Mason, 2003; Lavigne et al., 2000; Drewes, Nielsen, Arendt-Nielsen, Birket-Smith, & Hansen, 1997). Thus, the quality of sleep could be reduced by the presence of moderate to severe pain. Another explanation is that sleep disturbance causes or exacerbates chronic pain. This line of thinking is supported by studies demonstrating that sleep deprivation in healthy subjects can lead to painful symptoms and enhanced pain sensitivity. Moldofsky (Moldofsky & Scarisbrick, 1976; Moldofsky, Scarisbrick, England, & Smythe, 1975) first reported this phenomenon when he deprived healthy subjects of Stage 4 sleep (i.e., non-rapid eye movement deep sleep), and this produced pain, increased tenderness to palpation and mood symptoms similar to those seen in patients with musculoskeletal pain. More recently, Lentz, Landis, Rothermel, & Shaver (1999) reported that slow-wave sleep disruption lowered the mechanical pain threshold and produced fatigue and discomfort among middle-age women. Another experiment found that total sleep deprivation, but not slow-wave sleep interruption, lowered the mechanical pain threshold among healthy males; however, no effects on thermal pain perception emerged (Onen, Alloui, Gross, Eschallier, & Dubray, 2001). Another group of investigators showed no effect of slow-wave sleep interruption on pressure pain thresholds or pain symptoms (Older et al., 1998). Thus, sleep disruption alone may or may not produce pain-related symptoms and heightened pain sensitivity.

Another explanatory mechanism is that some third variable causes or maintains both chronic pain and sleep disturbance. For example, anxiety and depression are associated with insomnia and pain-related symptoms and could be an underlying cause of both. Also, as previously discussed, serotonin is important in regulating both sleep and pain; therefore, altered serotonin function could cause both conditions. Cognitive factors may also contribute to sleep disturbance associated with chronic pain. Smith and colleagues reported that pre-sleep cognitive arousal and thoughts related to pain and environmental stimuli predict sleep difficulties among patients with chronic pain

(Smith, Perlis, Carmody, Smith, & Giles, 2001; Smith, Perlis, Smith, Giles, & Carmody, 2000).

Regardless of the mechanisms underlying sleep disturbance in chronic pain, improving sleep among pain patients is an important treatment goal. Although pharmacotherapy is often utilized for this purpose, cognitive-behavioral treatments appear to be equally effective for management of insomnia (Edinger, Wohlgemuth, Radtke, Marsh, & Quillian, 2001; Smith et al., 2002; Murtagh & Greenwood, 1995). Among patients with chronic pain, uncontrolled and controlled trials indicate that behavioral treatment of insomnia is effective (Currie, Wilson, Pontefract, & de Laplante, 2000; Morin, Kowatch, & Wade, 1989). Moreover, patients whose sleep improved after insomnia treatment also reported reduced emotional distress and pain-related disability (Currie, Wilson, & Curran, 2002). Thus, successful treatment of insomnia may produce more general clinical benefits for patients with chronic pain.

social learning: Social learning, also known as vicarious or observational learning, refers to cognitive or behavioral changes acquired through observing others. As previously discussed (*see* FAMILY), individuals with a family history of pain are at increased risk for clinical pain and demonstrate enhanced sensitivity to experimental pain. Social learning could contribute to these familial influences on pain. Specifically, prior exposure to familial pain models may provide opportunities for incorporating pain-related responses into one's behavioral repertoire. Indeed, one study reported that among patients with a family history of pain, postoperative pain was greater for those who reported that their familial pain models had poor pain tolerance compared to those with pain-tolerant family members (Bachiocco, Scesi, Morselli, & Carli, 1993). In a laboratory study, female subjects exposed to pain-tolerant models demonstrated less sensitivity to pain and lower physiological responses to pain compared to controls (Craig & Prkachin, 1978). Thus, the type of pain models to which individuals are exposed can influence the subsequent experience of pain. This has important implications for pain treatment. Specifically, patients undergoing rehabilitation may benefit substantially from exposure to other patients coping effectively with pain and mastering functional tasks.

social support: No single definition of social support has been accepted, but it generally refers to the presence of others who provide emotional, material, informational, and behavioral support. Social support includes not only the number of social contacts and size of one's social network, but also the quality of social relationships and an individual's satisfaction with his or her social support. A robust literature indicates that better social support is associated with improved psychological and physical health (Taylor & Seeman, 1999; Taylor et al., 2000); however, the role of social support in adjustment to chronic pain is more complex. Specifically, as previously discussed (*see* FAMILY), spousal solicitousness, which may be construed as a form of social support, and patients' ratings of satisfaction with social support generally predict increased pain and disability among patients with chronic pain (Fillingim, Doleys, Edwards, & Lowery, 2003; Flor, Kerns, & Turk, 1987; Gil, Keefe, Crisson, & Van Dalfsen, 1987; Lousberg, Schmidt, & Groenman, 1992). However, the relationship between social support and pain-related adjustment has not been uniformly discouraging. For example, although perceived spousal solicitousness was positively associated with pain intensity among low back pain patients, the association was negative among patients with sickle-cell disease and arthritis (Anderson & Rehm, 1984). Moreover, among patients treated in a chronic pain-management program, higher pain-relevant social support predicted greater pain and disability; however, for patients with low problem-solving skills, high levels of social support were associated with decreased depression (Kerns, Rosenberg, & Otis, 2002). In a recent longitudinal study, lower perceived social support was associated with a greater increase in pain and functional disability over a five-year period in patients with rheumatoid arthritis (Evers, Kraaimaat, Geenen, Jacobs, & Bijlsma, 2003).

The most reasonable interpretation of these data might be that some forms of social support (e.g., solicitousness) are associated with poorer pain-related adjustment, and more appropriate forms of social support (e.g., encouraging effective coping, distraction) may confer protective effects against pain and disability. Instructing patients and their significant others in how to produce the most beneficial forms of social support may lead to improved long-term outcomes.

somatization: The term somatization is used in at least two ways. First, Somatization Disorder is a specific psychiatric condition, and more generally, the term *somatization* refers to a heightened somatic awareness of and increased concern regarding physical symptoms. Somatization Disorder is characterized by recurrent somatic complaints involving multiple bodily systems. Specifically, there must be pain symptoms from at least four different sites or bodily functions, at least two gastrointestinal complaints, at least one sexual symptom, and a pseudoneurological symptom (American Psychiatric Association, 1994). These symptoms cannot be explained based on medical findings. The prevalence is .2 to 2 percent among women and less than .2 percent in men (American Psychiatric Association, 1994). In a more general sense, the term *somatization* refers to excessive somatic focus or awareness and enhanced concern regarding physical symptoms, sharing considerable overlap with the construct of hypervigilance. (*See* HYPERVIGILANCE.)

spousal responses: *See* FAMILY.

stages of change: The stages of change derive from the Transtheoretical Model of Health Behavior, which posits that individuals progress through five different stages when making changes in behavior (Prochaska, DiClemente, & Norcross, 1992; Prochaska & Velicer, 1997; Prochaska & DiClemente, 1983).

1. *Precontemplation:* individuals have no intention of changing their behavior and may not recognize the need for behavior change.
2. *Contemplation:* involves recognition of the need for behavior change but no efforts to change have yet been attempted.
3. *Preparation:* involves making plans to implement behavior change.
4. *Action:* the stage during which actual changes in behavior are made.
5. *Maintenance:* people attempt to sustain the changes they have made.

This model has been widely applied to health behavior change, including smoking cessation, other addictive behaviors, weight loss, and exercise (Prochaska et al., 1992; Prochaska & Velicer, 1997); however, only recently have the stages of change been applied to chronic pain management.

Kerns, Rosenberg, Jamison, Caudill, & Haythornthwaite (1997) proposed that the stages of change model is particularly relevant to conceptualizing patients' readiness to produce the behavior changes involved in self-management approaches to coping with their chronic pain. These investigators developed and validated the Pain Stages of Change Questionnaire (PSOCQ) to assess patients' readiness to learn new methods for self-management of their pain (Kerns et al., 1997). The PSOCQ assesses responses related to the following four different stages of readiness for change:

> *precontemplation* (e.g., "The best thing I can do is find a doctor who can figure out how to get rid of my pain once and for all")
> *contemplation* (e.g., "I have recently figured out that it's up to me to deal better with my pain")
> *action* (e.g., "I am developing new ways to cope with my pain")
> *maintenance* (e.g., "I use what I have learned to help keep my pain under control")

Several studies support the validity of the PSOCQ. For example, patients' perceived control over pain and their reports of active coping correlate positively with the action and maintenance scales and negatively with the precontemplation scale of the PSOCQ (Kerns et al., 1997). Also, chronic pain patients who completed self-management treatment had higher pretreatment scores on contemplation and lower scores on precontemplation compared to noncompleters, suggesting that readiness to change predicts treatment compliance (Kerns & Rosenberg, 2000). Moreover, treatment completers showed significant increases in action and maintenance scores pre- to post-treatment, and these increases were associated with decreased pain behavior, depression, disability, and pain severity. Other researchers have provided additional evidence for the utility of the PSOCQ (Glenn & Burns, 2003; Jensen, Nielson, Turner, Romano, & Hill, 2003); however, some findings have questioned its factor structure, ability to accurately classify patients into stages, and applicability to non–pain-clinic samples (Habib, Morrissey, & Helmes, 2003; Strong, Westbury, Smith,

McKenzie, & Ryan, 2002; Jensen, Nielson, Romano, Hill, & Turner, 2000). Nonetheless, the application of the stages of change model to chronic pain management has intuitive appeal and may provide valuable information that can be used to tailor treatment and enhance outcomes.

stress: Stress can be defined as any demand placed upon an organism to adapt. Stress is often operationalized in terms of the occurrence of life events, and several instruments are available to assess such events. Holmes and Rahe (1967) developed the Social Readjustment Rating Scale, which lists 43 life events from most (death of spouse) to least (minor violations of the law) stressful, and subjects endorse the events that they have experienced over a specified period of time (e.g., the past six months). In order to assess more common, everyday stressful life events, Lazarus and colleagues developed the Hassles Scale (Kanner, Coyne, Schaefer, & Lazarus, 1981), on which subjects indicate which of 117 different hassles they have experienced during the past month and then rate the severity of each endorsed hassle. Other measures of recent life events and perceived stress have also been developed (Kohn, Lafreniere, & Gurevich, 1990; Kohn & Macdonald, 1992).

Voluminous data indicate that high levels of life stress are associated with chronic pain. For example, patients with chronic pain report more recent life events compared to pain-free controls, and high levels of stress are associated with more severe symptoms and poorer pain-related adjustment (Beaton, Egan, Nakagawa Kogan, & Morrison, 1991; Heim, Ehlert, Hanker, & Hellhammer, 1999; Lampe et al., 1998; Nahit, Pritchard, Cherry, Silman, & Macfarlane, 2001; Okifuji & Turk, 2002). Also, psychosocial stress appears to increase risk for developing pain (Kopec, Sayre, & Esdaile, 2004; Linton, 2000; Nahit et al., 2003). Several mechanisms whereby stress could adversely affect patients with chronic pain have been found. First, stress is associated with biological changes that can exacerbate pain. For example, laboratory studies demonstrate that experimentally induced stress can produce increased muscle tension at painful body sites, which could increase clinical pain (Flor & Turk, 1989; Flor, Birbaumer, Schulte, & Roos, 1991). Also, stress produces sympathetic activation, which can aggravate pain conditions with a sympathetic component (e.g., complex regional pain syndrome), and stress-induced vasoconstriction can exacerbate vascular and/or ischemic pain conditions (e.g., Raynaud's, angina, migraine). Psychological responses to stress, including emotional distress and negative thinking, can also increase pain severity. It is also important to recognize that the presence of significant life stress may overtax coping resources such that the individual is no longer able to cope effectively with chronic pain.

The relationship between stress and pain can be bidirectional. For example, in both animals and humans, acute stress can produce analgesia (Akil, Young, Walker, & Watson, 1986; Flor & Grusser, 1999; Madden, Akil, Patrick, & Barchas, 1977; Watkins et al., 1984). However, recent studies in rodents indicate that repeated bouts of stress lead to prolonged hyperalgesia (Quintero et al., 2000, 2003). Thus, stress produces wide-ranging physiological and psychological effects, which can affect the experience of pain in complex ways. The persistent and elevated levels of psychosocial stress faced by patients with chronic pain exacerbates clinical pain, and interventions to enhance stress coping (e.g., cognitive-behavioral treatment) are an important component of treatment.

suffering: Suffering is a state of distress that occurs when the integrity of the person is threatened (Cassell, 1999). Pain-related suffering refers to the overall personal distress that an individual experiences in the context of pain, which includes physical, emotional, existential, and social aspects (Chapman & Gavrin, 1999). Chronic pain is typically associated with considerable suffering, given its adverse affects on virtually all areas of life. The amelioration of suffering is what patients seek most, and this requires viewing the patient as a whole person, taking into account his or her personal history and the social context in which the suffering occurs (Cassell, 1999).

suicide: Suicide is the eleventh leading cause of death in the United States, and the third leading cause of death for people age 15 to 24 (Centers for Disease Control and Prevention, 2003). In 2000, suicide resulted in 29,350 deaths, more than homicide. Males are four times more likely to commit suicide than females, though females are more likely to attempt suicide (Centers for Disease Control and Prevention, 2003). Chronic pain appears to increase suicide risk (Fishbain, 1999; Fisher, Haythornthwaite, Heinberg, Clark, & Reed, 2001), and pain is a factor in physician-assisted suicide (Roscoe, Malphurs, Dragovic,

& Cohen, 2003). This may be partly due to the increased prevalence of depression among chronic pain patients, because cognitive/affective factors (e.g., hopelessness, emotional distress, impulsivity) remain the strongest predictors of suicide risk (Conner, Duberstein, Conwell, Seidlitz, & Caine, 2001; Fawcett, Busch, Jacobs, Kravitz, & Fogg, 1997). These findings illustrate the need to assess suicidality among patients with chronic pain and to appropriately intervene when suicidal intent is present.

T **temporal summation:** Temporal summation of pain, in general, refers to increased perception of a stimulus with prolonged stimulus duration. A specific form of temporal summation occurs when brief, repetitive suprathreshold stimuli are administered rapidly, which produces increasing pain even though the stimulus intensity is constant (Price, Hu, Dubner, & Gracely, 1977; Price, Mao, Frenk, & Mayer, 1994; Vierck, Cannon, Fry, Maixner, & Whitsel, 1997). Temporal summation appears to result from hyperactivity in second-order neurons, due to activation of the NMDA-receptor by excitatory neuropeptides released from primary afferents, and it is reversed by NMDA receptor antagonists such as dextromethorphan and ketamine (Arendt-Nielsen, Nielsen, Petersen-Felix, Schnider, & Zbinden, 1996; Price et al., 1994). Similar mechanisms of neuronal plasticity may be involved in the central sensitization observed in many clinical pain conditions. Enhanced temporal summation of pain was demonstrated in neuropathic pain conditions (Eide, 2000) as well as nociceptive pain conditions such as fibromyalgia (Staud, Vierck, Cannon, Mauderli, & Price, 2001) and temporomandibular disorders (Maixner, Fillingim, Sigurdsson, Kincaid, & Silva, 1998). Temporal summation can also be influenced by individual difference variables, such as gender (Fillingim, Maixner, Kincaid, & Silva, 1998; Sarlani & Greenspan, 2002) and age (Edwards & Fillingim, 2001), both of which are associated with elevated risk for experiencing clinical pain. Moreover, recent evidence suggests that psychosocial variables, such as anxiety and willingness to report pain, may contribute to temporal summation of pain (Robinson, Wise, Gagnon, Fillingim, & Price, 2004). Thus, temporal summation represents a clinically relevant phenomenon, whose systematic investigation in the laboratory may elucidate mechanisms contributing to certain chronic pain disorders.

temporomandibular disorders: Temporomandibular disorders (TMD) represent a group of conditions characterized by pain and dysfunction in the temporomandibular joint (TMJ) and/or the surrounding muscles (Dworkin, 1999). Signs and symptoms of TMD include joint sounds, such as clicking and crepitus during mandibular motion, limited mouth opening, pain on palpation of masticatory muscles, and pain on function. These disorders are common, with a prevalence of approximately 12 percent in the U.S. population (Dworkin et al., 1990; LeResche, 1997). The female-to-male ratio in the community ranges from 1.2 to 2.6, with an average of two (Drangsholt & LeResche, 1999). Dworkin (1999) noted that TMD patients display many similarities to patients with other chronic pain syndromes, including: low correspondence between subjective symptoms and objective pathophysiological findings; maladaptive behaviors that negatively impact symptoms (e.g., clenching and other parafunctions); clinically significant psychological distress; pain interferes with occupational, social and/or interpersonal function; and excessive use of the health care system by a proportion of patients. Thus, TMD is a common and often disabling chronic pain disorder.

The etiopathogenesis of TMD remains unknown, but some investigators proposed that alterations in central pain modulation play an important role in the etiology and maintenance of TMD (Maixner, Sigurdsson, Fillingim, Lundeen, & Booker, 1995). Some evidence suggests enhanced sensitivity to pain primarily in the facial muscles among TMD patients (Svensson, List, & Hector, 2001; Svensson, Arendt-Nielsen, Nielsen, & Larsen, 1995); however, others demonstrated greater pain sensitivity in body regions outside the painful area (Maixner, Fillingim, Booker, & Sigurdsson, 1995; Malow, Grimm, & Olson, 1980), including more pronounced temporal summation of thermal pain (Molin, Edman, & Schalling, 1973; Maixner, Fillingim, Sigurdsson, Kincaid, & Silva, 1998). Lower tolerance of ischemic arm pain was associated with enhanced clinical pain (Fillingim, Maixner, Kincaid, Sigurdsson, & Harris, 1996). Taken together, these findings provide strong evidence that TMD is characterized by enhanced sensitivity to painful stimuli.

Psychosocial factors are important in TMD. Indeed, TMD cases exhibit significantly greater psychological distress than pain-free controls (Velly, Gornitsky, & Philippe, 2003; Pedroni, De Oliveira, & Guaratini, 2003; Macfarlane, Gray, Kincey, & Worthington, 2001; Rollman

& Gillespie, 2000), and TMD patients whose pain is primarily muscular in origin show greater psychological dysfunction compared to TMD patients with joint pain (Huang, LeResche, Critchlow, Martin, & Drangsholt, 2002; Lindroth, Schmidt, & Carlson, 2002; Auerbach, Laskin, Frantsve, & Orr, 2001; Kight, Gatchel, & Wesley, 1999). Psychological factors, such as depression, anxiety, and catastrophizing, are associated with more severe pain-related symptoms (Turner, Dworkin, Mancl, Huggins, & Truelove, 2001; Madland, Feinmann, & Newman, 2000; Rollman & Gillespie, 2000), and psychosocial dysfunction predicts treatment-seeking and poorer long-term prognosis in TMD (Auerbach et al., 2001; Epker, Gatchel, & Ellis, 1999; Epker & Gatchel, 2000; Garofalo, Gatchel, Wesley, & Ellis, 1998; Ohrbach & Dworkin, 1998). Moreover, cognitive-behavioral treatment is effective for reducing pain, disability, and psychological distress in TMD patients (Dworkin et al., 1994; Flor & Birbaumer, 1993; Mishra, Gatchel, & Gardea, 2000; Oakley et al., 1994; Sherman & Turk, 2001; Stam, McGrath, & Brooke, 1984). Thus, TMD, as with many other chronic pain disorders, is associated with increased psychological dysfunction, and psychological interventions are effective for improving pain-related adjustment.

treatment outcome: The assessment of treatment outcome is an important and complex issue in evaluating the effectiveness of interventions for pain. Choosing among the multiple methods available for assessing pain is challenging enough (*see* PAIN ASSESSMENT); however, multiple outcomes in addition to pain reduction are of clinical importance in treating patients with chronic pain. In this regard, the Initiative on Methods, Measurement, and Pain Assessment in Clinical Trials (IMMPACT) recently developed consensus recommendations for outcomes assessment in chronic pain clinical trials (Dworkin et al., 2005). This expert panel identified the following six core outcome domains that should be assessed in clinical trials involving patients with chronic pain:

1. pain,
2. physical functioning,
3. emotional functioning,
4. participant ratings of improvement and satisfaction with treatment,

5. symptoms and adverse events, and
6. participant disposition (e.g., adherence to the treatment regimen and reasons for premature withdrawal from the trial).

Thus, assessment of treatment outcomes should include multiple clinical end points, and effective interventions should lead to improvements across each of these important symptom domains.

validity: The term validity refers to the extent to which a measurement method assesses the construct it purports to measure, and validity is the most important factor in determining the utility of a measure (Jensen, 2003). As previously noted (*see* RELIABILITY), a measure cannot be valid unless it is also reliable; however, a reliable measure can be invalid. Validity is conceptualized with respect to a particular end point or outcome; that is, a measure is not valid in general, rather it is valid for a specific purpose. The three most important forms of validity are content validity, construct validity, and criterion-related validity (Jensen, 2003). Content validity refers to whether a measure assesses as a representative sample of the domain of interest (Anastasi, 1982). For example, a measure of pain disability that only measured occupational function and ignored other important domains such as social or leisure activities or activities of daily living would have poor content validity. Content validity is an essential component of test development and is usually verified using expert analysis (Jensen, 2003). Construct validity is the extent to which an instrument measures a theoretical or conceptual construct (Anastasi, 1982). That is, to what degree does the Pain Anxiety and Symptom Scale assess the construct of pain-related anxiety? This is typically determined by correlating the instrument with other known measures of the construct. Also, factor analysis is used in determining construct validity (for more information see Jensen, 2003). In determining construct validity, it is also important that an instrument does not correlate with measures of unrelated constructs (Anastasi, 1982). Criterion-related validity is the extent to which a measure is associated with important end points. An example of criterion-related validity would be a correlation between pain-related anxiety and pain-related disability (the criterion). Clinicians should rely on assessment instruments that have been well validated, and pain researchers should present evidence of the validity of the measures used in their investigations.

visual analog scales: *See* PAIN ASSESSMENT.

 Waddell signs: The Waddell Signs (or inorganic signs) are behavioral responses to physical examination that are thought to reflect abnormal illness behavior (Waddell, McCulloch, Kummel, & Venner, 1980). The eight original signs include the following:

- superficial tenderness
- nonanatomic tenderness
- pain in response to axial loading (i.e., vertical downward pressure on the top of the head when standing)
- back pain in response to simulated rotation (i.e., simultaneous rotation of the shoulders and pelvis)
- improved straight leg raise response when distracted
- weakness that is not consistent with normal neurologic function
- sensory loss that does not follow a dermatomal pattern
- "overreaction" to the physical examination (Waddell et al., 1980)

These signs can be reliably assessed, and are correlated with important clinical measures, such as disability, clinical history, and psychosocial factors (Main & Waddell, 1998; Novy et al., 1998). The signs were originally developed to detect a *pattern* of abnormal responding to physical examination, and overinterpretation of individual signs was cautioned against (Waddell, Main, Morris, Di Paola, & Gray, 1984; Waddell et al., 1980). Unfortunately, the signs have been misinterpreted and misused over the years, and considerable confusion exists as to what these signs mean (Fishbain et al., 2003; Main & Waddell, 1998). The most troubling inappropriate use of the signs has been the interpretation that they reflect malingering or conscious symptom exaggeration by patients (Fishbain et al., 2003; Main & Waddell, 1998). The developers of the Waddell signs were careful to present them as a source of behavioral data that must be interpreted in the context of additional clinical history, as well as medical and psychological testing (Main & Waddell, 1998; Waddell et al., 1984; Waddell et al., 1980). A recent meta-analysis of research using the Waddell signs concluded that the signs are associated with decreased function, higher pain severity, and poorer outcomes from nonsurgical treatment (Fishbain et al., 2003). However, the authors found no evidence that the Waddell signs were associated with psychological distress or secondary gain and they concluded that the signs likely reflect organic phenomena and should not be used to discriminate organic from nonorganic pain conditions. Thus, the Waddell signs are commonly used behavioral responses to physical examination; however, their clinical value remains somewhat unclear.

workers' compensation: Chronic pain accounts for a large proportion of worker's compensation claims, and low back pain is the leading cause of occupational injury in developed countries (Battie & Bigos, 1991; Guo, Tanaka, Halperin, & Cameron, 1999). Approximately 10 percent of the cases absorb more than 80 percent of the cost for low back pain because of their chronicity (Hashemi, Webster, & Clancy, 1998; Volinn, Van Koevering, & Loeser, 1991; Murphy & Courtney, 2000). Historically, clinicians believed that patients receiving workers' compensation (i.e., pain-contingent disability payments) were more likely to exaggerate pain-related symptoms and would show poorer outcomes from treatment; thus the term "compensation neurosis." These impressions involved mixed evidence. For example, several studies indicate that patients receiving compensation report greater pain and disability and show poorer outcomes from treatments (Fow, Dorris, Sittig, & Smith-Seemiller, 2002; Groth-Marnat & Fletcher, 2000; Rainville, Sobel, Hartigan, & Wright, 1997; Carron, DeGood, & Tait, 1985; Greenough & Fraser, 1989; Fredrickson, Trief, VanBeveren, Yuan, & Baum, 1988). In contrast, other studies suggested that compensation is not associated with pretreatment pain or disability and that compensation patients respond equally well to treatments (Trabin, Rader, & Cummings, 1987; Jamison, Matt, & Parris, 1988; Leavitt, Garron, McNeill, & Whisler, 1982; Dworkin, Handlin, Richlin, Brand, & Vannucci, 1985).

Thus, whether workers' compensation affects clinical features and long-term prognosis is a complicated issue. Work-related factors may moderate the relationship between compensation status and clinical variables. Cross-sectional and prospective studies demonstrated that occupational factors, such as job dissatisfaction, work stress, and physical demands of work, predict the presence of pain and the chronicity of pain and disability (Schultz et al., 2002; Fransen et al., 2002; Cole, Ibrahim, Shannon, Scott, & Eyles, 2001; Miranda, Viikari-Juntura, Martikainen, Takala, & Riihimaki, 2001; Bigos et al., 1992; Krause, Dasinger, Deegan, Rudolph, & Brand, 2001; Nahit, Pritchard, Cherry, Silman, & Macfarlane, 2001). It seems plausible that such adverse workplace factors may be particularly associated with poor prognosis among patients receiving workers' compensation for chronic pain. Thus, the presence of workers' compensation and other work-related factors are important considerations in the assessment and treatment of patients with chronic pain; however, these factors do not uniformly predict poor motivation and poor prognosis.

References

Introduction

Dworkin, R. H., & Breitbart, W. S. (2004). *Psychosocial aspects of pain: A handbook for health care providers.* Seattle: IASP Press.

Gatchel, R. J., & Turk, D. C. (1999). *Psychosocial factors in pain.* New York: Guilford Press.

Hadjistavropoulos, T., & Craig, K. D. (2004). *Pain: Psychological perspectives.* Mahwah, NJ: Lawrence Erlbaum Associates.

Price, D. D. (2000). *Psychological mechanisms of pain and analgesia.* Seattle: IASP Press.

Turk, D. C., & Gatchel, R. J. (2002). *Psychological approaches to pain management: A practitioner's handbook.* New York: Guilford Press.

Abuse

Alexander, R. W., Bradley, L. A., Alarcon, G. S., Triana-Alexander, M., Aaron, L. A., Alberts, K. R., Martin, M. Y., & Stewart, K. E. (1998). Sexual and physical abuse in women with fibromyalgia: Association with outpatient health care utilization and pain medication usage. *Arthritis Care & Research, 11,* 102-115.

Bendixen, M., Muus, K. M., & Schei, B. (1994). The impact of child sexual abuse— A study of a random sample of Norwegian students. *Child Abuse & Neglect, 18,* 837-847.

Boisset-Pioro, M. H., Esdaile, J. M., & Fitzcharles, M. (1995). Sexual and physical abuse in women with fibromyalgia syndrome. *Arthritis and Rheumatism, 38,* 235-241.

Domino, J. V., & Haber, J. D. (1987). Prior physical and sexual abuse in women with chronic headache: Clinical correlates. *Headache, 27,* 310-314.

Drossman, D. A., Leserman, J., Nachman, G., Li, Z., Gluck, H., Toomey, T. C., & Mitchell, M. (1990). Sexual and physical abuse in women with functional or organic gastrointestinal disorders. *Annals of Internal Medicine, 113,* 828-833.

Fillingim, R. B., & Edwards, R. R. Is self-reported childhood abuse history associated with pain perception among healthy young women and men? *Clinical Journal of Pain* (in press).

Fillingim, R. B., Maixner, W., Sigurdsson, A., & Kincaid, S. (1997). Sexual and physical abuse history in subjects with temporomandibular disorders: Relationship to clinical variables, pain sensitivity, and psychologic factors. *Journal of Orofacial Pain, 11*[1], 48-57.

Fillingim, R. B., Wilkinson, C. S., & Powell, T. (1999). Self-reported abuse history and pain complaints among healthy young adults. *Clinical Journal of Pain, 15,* 85-91.

Goldberg, R. T. (1994). Childhood abuse, depression, and chronic pain. *Clinical Journal of Pain, 10,* 277-281.

Green, C. R., Flowe-Valencia, H., Rosenblum, L., & Tait, A. R. (1999). Do physical and sexual abuse differentially affect chronic pain states in women? *Journal of Pain and Symptom Management, 18,* 420-426.

Green, C. R., Flowe-Valencia, H., Rosenblum, L., & Tait, A. R. (2001). The role of childhood and adulthood abuse among women presenting for chronic pain management. *Clinical Journal of Pain, 17,* 359-364.

Lautenbacher, S., Rollman, G. B., & McCain, G. A. (1994). Multi-method assessment of experimental and clinical pain in patients with fibromyalgia. *Pain, 59,* 45-53.

Leserman, J., Drossman, D. A., Li, Z., Toomey, T. C., Nachman, G., & Glogau, L. (1996). Sexual and physical abuse history in gastroenterology practice: How types of abuse impact health status. *Psychosomatic Medicine, 58,* 4-15.

Linton, S. J. (1997). A population-based study of the relationship between sexual abuse and back pain: Establishing a link. *Pain, 73,* 47-53.

Linton, S. J. (2002). A prospective study of the effects of sexual or physical abuse on back pain. *Pain, 96,* 347-351.

Linton, S. J., Larden, M., & Gillow, A. M. (1996). Sexual abuse and chronic musculoskeletal pain: Prevalence and psychological factors. *Clinical Journal of Pain, 12,* 215-221.

Maixner, W., Fillingim, R., Booker, D., & Sigurdsson, A. (1995). Sensitivity of patients with painful temporomandibular disorders to experimentally evoked pain. *Pain, 63,* 341-351.

Nickel, R., Egle, U. T., & Hardt, J. (2002). Are childhood adversities relevant in patients with chronic low back pain? *European Journal of Pain, 6,* 221-228.

Raphael, K. G., Widom, C. S., & Lange, G. (2001). Childhood victimization and pain in adulthood: A prospective investigation. *Pain, 92,* 283-293.

Scarinci, I. C., McDonald-Haile, J., Bradley, L. A., & Richter, J. E. (1994). Altered pain perception and psychosocial features among women with gastrointestinal disorders and history of abuse: A preliminary model. *American Journal of Medicine, 97,* 108-118.

Taylor, M. L., Trotter, D. R., & Csuka, M. E. (1995). The prevalence of sexual abuse in women with fibromyalgia. *Arthritis and Rheumatism, 38,* 229-234.

Toomey, T. C., Seville, J. L., Mann, J. D., Abashian, S. W., & Grant, J. (1995). Relationship of sexual and physical abuse to pain description, coping, psychological distress, and health-care utilization in a chronic pain sample. *Clinical Journal of Pain, 11,* 307-315.

Verne, G. N., Robinson, M. E., & Price, D. D. (2001). Hypersensitivity to visceral and cutaneous pain in the irritable bowel syndrome. *Pain, 93,* 7-14.

Walker, E. A., Katon, W. J., Neraas, K., Jemelka, R. P., & Massoth, D. (1992). Dissociation in women with chronic pelvic pain. *American Journal of Psychiatry, 149,* 534-537.

Walker, E. A., Keegan, D., Gardner, G., Sullivan, M., Bernstein, D., & Katon, W. J. (1997). Psychosocial factors in fibromyalgia compared with rheumatoid arthritis: II. Sexual, physical, and emotional abuse and neglect. *Psychosomatic Medicine, 59,* 572-577.

Walling, M. K., Reiter, R. C., O'Hara, M. W., Milburn, A. K., Lilly, G., & Vincent, S. D. (1994). Abuse history and chronic pain in women: I. Prevalences of sexual abuse and physical abuse. *Obstetrics & Gynecology, 84,* 193-199.

Whitehead, W. E., Crowell, M. D., Davidoff, A. L., Palsson, O. S., & Schuster, M. M. (1997). Pain from rectal distension in women with irritable bowel syndrome: Relationship to sexual abuse. *Digestive Diseases & Sciences, 42,* 796-804.

Wurtele, S. K., Kaplan, G. M., & Keairnes, M. (1990). Childhood sexual abuse among chronic pain patients. *Clinical Journal of Pain, 6,* 110-113.

Acceptance

McCracken, L. M. (1998). Learning to live with the pain: Acceptance of pain predicts adjustment in persons with chronic pain. *Pain, 74,* 21-27.

McCracken, L. M., & Eccleston, C. (2003). Coping or acceptance: What to do about chronic pain? *Pain, 105,* 197-204.

McCracken, L. M., Spertus, I. L., Janeck, A. S., Sinclair, D., & Wetzel, F. T. (1999). Behavioral dimensions of adjustment in persons with chronic pain: Pain-related anxiety and acceptance. *Pain, 80,* 283-289.

Risdon, A., Eccleston, C., Crombez, G., & McCracken, L. (2003). How can we learn to live with pain? A Q-methodological analysis of the diverse understandings of acceptance of chronic pain. *Social Science & Medicine, 56,* 375-386.

Viane, I., Crombez, G., Eccleston, C., Poppe, C., Devulder, J., Van Houdenhove, B., & De Corte, W. (2003). Acceptance of pain is an independent predictor of mental well-being in patients with chronic pain: Empirical evidence and reappraisal. *Pain, 106,* 65-72.

Acute pain

Bandura, A., Cioffi, D., Taylor, C. B., & Brouillard, M. E. (1988). Perceived self-efficacy in coping with cognitive stressors and opioid activation. *Journal of Personality and Social Psychology, 55,* 479-488.

Caumo, W., Schmidt, A. P., Schneider, C. N., Bergmann, J., Iwamoto, C. W., Adamatti, L. C., Bandeira, D., & Ferreira, M. B. (2002). Preoperative predictors of moderate to intense acute postoperative pain in patients undergoing abdominal surgery. *Acta Anaesthesiologica Scandinavica, 46,* 1265-1271.

France, C. R., France, J. L., al'Absi, M., Ring, C., & McIntyre, D. (2002). Catastrophizing is related to pain ratings, but not nociceptive flexion reflex threshold. *Pain, 99,* 459-463.

Gil, K. M., Ginsberg, B., Muir, M., Sykes, D., & Williams, D. A. (1990). Patient-controlled analgesia in postoperative pain: The relation of psychological factors to pain and analgesic use. *Clinical Journal of Pain, 2,* 137-142.

Luebbert, K., Dahme, B., & Hasenbring, M. (2001). The effectiveness of relaxation training in reducing treatment-related symptoms and improving emotional adjustment in acute non-surgical cancer treatment: A meta-analytical review. *Psycho-Oncology, 10,* 490-502.

Montgomery, G. H., David, D., Winkel, G., Silverstein, J. H., & Bovbjerg, D. H. (2002). The effectiveness of adjunctive hypnosis with surgical patients: A meta-analysis. *Anesthesia Analgesia, 94,* 1639-1645.

Nelson, F. V., Zimmerman, L., Barnason, S., Nieveen, J., & Schmaderer, M. (1998). The relationship and influence of anxiety on postoperative pain in the coronary artery bypass graft patient. *Journal of Pain and Symptom Management, 15,* 102-109.

Patterson, D. R., & Jensen, M. P. (2003). Hypnosis and clinical pain. *Psychology Bulletin, 129,* 495-521.

Perry, F., Parker, R. K., White, P. F., & Clifford, P. A. (1994). Role of psychological factors in postoperative pain control and recovery with patient-controlled analgesia. *Clinical Journal of Pain, 10,* 57-63.

Pollo, A., Amanzio, M., Arslanian, A., Casadio, C., Maggi, G., & Benedetti, F. (2001). Response expectancies in placebo analgesia and their clinical relevance. *Pain, 93,* 77-84.

Villemure, C., & Bushnell, M. C. (2002). Cognitive modulation of pain: How do attention and emotion influence pain processing? *Pain, 95,* 195-199.

Williams, D. A. (2004). Evaluating acute pain. In R. H. Dworkin & W. S. Breitbart (Eds.), *Psychosocial aspects of pain: A handbook for health care providers* (pp. 79-96). Seattle: IASP Press.

Addiction

American Psychiatric Association (1994). *Diagnostic and statistical manual of mental disorders: DSM-IV* (4th ed.). Washington, DC: American Psychiatric Association.

Bendtsen, P., Hensing, G., Ebeling, C., & Schedin, A. (1999). What are the qualities of dilemmas experienced when prescribing opioids in general practice? *Pain, 82,* 89-96.

Compton, P., & Athanasos, P. (2003). Chronic pain, substance abuse and addiction. *Nursing Clinics of North America, 38,* 525-537.

Fishbain, D. A., Rosomoff, H. L., & Rosomoff, R. S. (1992). Drug abuse, dependence, and addiction in chronic pain patients. *Clinical Journal of Pain, 8,* 77-85.

Gilron, I., & Bailey, J. M. (2003). Trends in opioid use for chronic neuropathic pain: A survey of patients pursuing enrollment in clinical trials. *Canadian Journal of Anesthesia, 50,* 42-47.

Gilron, I., Bailey, J., Weaver, D. F., & Houlden, R. L. (2002). Patients' attitudes and prior treatments in neuropathic pain: A pilot study. *Pain Research & Management, 7*, 199-203.

Joranson, D. E., Ryan, K. M., Gilson, A. M., & Dahl, J. L. (2000). Trends in medical use and abuse of opioid analgesics. *Journal of the American Medical Association, 283*, 1710-1714.

Morley-Forster, P. K., Clark, A. J., Speechley, M., & Moulin, D. E. (2003). Attitudes toward opioid use for chronic pain: A Canadian physician survey. *Pain Research & Management, 8*, 189-194.

Moulin, D. E., Clark, A. J., Speechley, M., & Morley-Forster, P. K. (2002). Chronic pain in Canada—Prevalence, treatment, impact and the role of opioid analgesia. *Pain Research & Management, 7*, 179-184.

Passik, S. D., & Weinreb, H. J. (2000). Managing chronic nonmalignant pain: Overcoming obstacles to the use of opioids. *Advances in Therapy, 17*, 70-83.

Portenoy, R. K. (1996). Opioid therapy for chronic nonmalignant pain: A review of the critical issues. *Journal of Pain and Symptom Management, 11*, 203-217.

Potter, M., Schafer, S., Gonzalez-Mendez, E., Gjeltema, K., Lopez, A., Wu, J., Pedrin, R., Cozen, M., Wilson, R., Thom, D., & Croughan-Minihane, M. (2001). Opioids for chronic nonmalignant pain. Attitudes and practices of primary care physicians in the UCSF/Stanford Collaborative Research Network. University of California, San Francisco. *Journal of Family Practice, 50*, 145-151.

Savage, S. R., Joranson, D. E., Covington, E. C., Schnoll, S. H., Heit, H. A., & Gilson, A. M. (2003). Definitions related to the medical use of opioids: Evolution towards universal agreement. *Journal of Pain and Symptom Management, 26*, 655-667.

Weiner, D. K., & Rudy, T. E. (2002). Attitudinal barriers to effective treatment of persistent pain in nursing home residents. *Journal of the American Geriatrics Society, 50*, 2035-2040.

Weissman, D. E., & Haddox, J. D. (1989). Opioid pseudoaddiction—An iatrogenic syndrome. *Pain, 36*, 363-366.

Zacny, J., Bigelow, G., Compton, P., Foley, K., Iguchi, M., & Sannerud, C. (2003). College on Problems of Drug Dependence taskforce on prescription opioid non-medical use and abuse: Position statement. *Drug & Alcohol Dependence, 69*, 215-232.

Aging

Edwards, R. R., & Fillingim, R. B. (2001a). Age-associated differences in responses to noxious stimuli. *Journals of Gerontology Series A: Biological Sciences and Medical Sciences, 56*, M180-M185.

Edwards, R. R., & Fillingim, R. B. (2001b). Effects of age on temporal summation of thermal pain: Clinical relevance in healthy older and younger adults. *Journal of Pain, 2*, 307-317.

Edwards, R. R., Fillingim, R. B., & Ness, T. J. (2003). Age-related differences in endogenous pain modulation: A comparison of diffuse noxious inhibitory controls in healthy older and younger adults. *Pain, 101,* 155-165.

Gagliese, L., & Melzack, R. (1997). Chronic pain in elderly people. *Pain, 70,* 3-14.

Gibson, S. J., & Helme, R. D. (2001). Age-related differences in pain perception and report. *Clinics in Geriatric Medicine, 17,* 433-456.

Gibson, S. J., Katz, B., Corran, T. M., Farrell, M. J., & Helme, R. D. (1994). Pain in older persons. *Disability & Rehabilitation: An International Multidisciplinary Journal, 16,* 127-139.

Gureje, O., Simon, G. E., & Von Korff, M. (2001). A cross-national study of the course of persistent pain in primary care. *Pain, 92,* 195-200.

Harkins, S. W. (1996). Geriatric pain. Pain perceptions in the old. *Clinics in Geriatric Medicine, 12,* 435-459.

Harkins, S. W., & Chapman, C. R. (1977). Age and sex differences in pain perception. In D. J. Anderson & B. Matthews (Eds.), *Pain in the trigeminal region* (pp. 435-441). Amsterdam: Elsevier.

Harkins, S. W., & Scott, R. B. (1996). Pain and presbyalgos. In J. E. Birren (Ed.), *Encyclopedia of gerontology: Age, aging, and the aged* (pp. 247-260). San Diego: Academic Press.

Helme, R. D., & Gibson, S. J. (2001). The epidemiology of pain in elderly people. *Clinics in Geriatric Medicine, 17,* 417-431.

Kendig, H., Browning, C. J., & Young, A. E. (2000). Impacts of illness and disability on the well-being of older people. *Disability and Rehabilitation, 22,* 15-22.

Scudds, R. J., & Robertson, J. M. (1998). Empirical evidence of the association between the presence of musculoskeletal pain and physical disability in community-dwelling senior citizens. *Pain, 75,* 229-235.

Verhaak, P. F., Kerssens, J. J., Dekker, J., Sorbi, M. J., & Bensing, J. M. (1998). Prevalence of chronic benign pain disorder among adults: A review of the literature. *Pain, 77,* 231-239.

Walsh, N. E., Schoenfeld, L., Ramamurthy, S., & Hoffman, J. (1989). Normative model for cold pressor test. *American Journal of Physical Medicine and Rehabilitation, 68,* 6-11.

Washington, L. L., Gibson, S. J., & Helme, R. D. (2000). Age-related differences in the endogenous analgesic response to repeated cold water immersion in human volunteers. *Pain, 89,* 89-96.

Alexithymia

Bagby, R. M., Parker, J. D., & Taylor, G. J. (1994). The twenty-item Toronto Alexithymia Scale—I. Item selection and cross-validation of the factor structure. *Journal of Psychosomatic Research, 38,* 23-32.

Bagby, R. M., Taylor, G. J., & Parker, J. D. (1994). The twenty-item Toronto Alexithymia Scale—II. Convergent, discriminant, and concurrent validity. *Journal of Psychosomatic Research, 38,* 33-40.

Lumley, M. A., Smith, J. A., & Longo, D. J. (2002). The relationship of alexithymia to pain severity and impairment among patients with chronic myofascial pain: Comparisons with self-efficacy, catastrophizing, and depression. *Journal of Psychosomatic Research, 53,* 823-830.

Lumley, M. A., Stettner, L., & Wehmer, F. (1996). How are alexithymia and physical illness linked? A review and critique of pathways. *Journal of Psychosomatic Research, 41,* 505-518.

Parker, J. D., Taylor, G. J., & Bagby, R. M. (2003). The 20-Item Toronto Alexithymia Scale. III. Reliability and factorial validity in a community population. *Journal of Psychosomatic Research, 55,* 269-275.

Porcelli, P., Taylor, G. J., Bagby, R. M., & De Carne, M. (1999). Alexithymia and functional gastrointestinal disorders. A comparison with inflammatory bowel disease. *Psychotherapy and Psychosomatics, 68,* 263-269.

Taylor, G. J., Bagby, R. M., & Parker, J. D. (2003). The 20-Item Toronto Alexithymia Scale. IV. Reliability and factorial validity in different languages and cultures. *Journal of Psychosomatic Research, 55,* 277-283.

Taylor, G. J., Ryan, D., & Bagby, R. M. (1985). Toward the development of a new self-report alexithymia scale. *Psychotherapy and Psychosomatics, 44,* 191-199.

Allodynia

Merskey, H., & Bogduk, N. (1994). *Classification of chronic pain* (2nd ed.). Seattle: IASP Press.

Alternative medicine

Astin, J. A. (1998). Why patients use alternative medicine: Results of a national study. *Journal of the American Medical Association, 279,* 1548-1553.

Cauffield, J. S. (2000). The psychosocial aspects of complementary and alternative medicine. *Pharmacotherapy, 20,* 1289-1294.

Smith, C. A., Collins, C. T., Cyna, A. M., & Crowther, C. A. (2003). Complementary and alternative therapies for pain management in labour. *The Cochrane Database of Systematic Reviews,* CD003521.

Snyder, M., & Wieland, J. (2003). Complementary and alternative therapies: What is their place in the management of chronic pain? *Nursing Clinics of North America, 38,* 495-508.

Soeken, K. L. (2004). Selected CAM therapies for arthritis-related pain: The evidence from systematic reviews. *Clinical Journal of Pain, 20,* 13-18.

Weintraub, M. I. (2003). Complementary and alternative methods of treatment of neck pain. *Physical Medicine and Rehabilitation Clinics of North America, 14,* viii, 659-674.

Analgesia

Merskey, H., & Bogduk, N. (1994). *Classification of chronic pain* (2nd ed.). Seattle: IASP Press.

Price, D. D. (2000). *Psychological mechanisms of pain and analgesia.* Seattle: IASP Press.

Anger

Bruehl, S., Chung, O. Y., & Burns, J. W. (2003). Differential effects of expressive anger regulation on chronic pain intensity in CRPS and non-CRPS limb pain patients. *Pain, 104,* 647-654.

Burns, J. W., Johnson, B. J., Devine, J., Mahoney, N., & Pawl, R. (1998). Anger management style and the prediction of treatment outcome among male and female chronic pain patients. *Behaviour Research and Therapy, 36,* 1051-1062.

Burns, J. W., Johnson, B. J., Mahoney, N., Devine, J., & Pawl, R. (1996). Anger management style, hostility and spouse responses: Gender differences in predictors of adjustment among chronic pain patients. *Pain, 64,* 445-453.

Burns, J. W., Kubilus, A., & Bruehl, S. (2003). Emotion induction moderates effects of anger management style on acute pain sensitivity. *Pain, 106,* 109-118.

Fernandez, E., & Turk, D. C. (1995). The scope and significance of anger in the experience of chronic pain. *Pain, 61,* 165-175.

Greenwood, K. A., Thurston, R., Rumble, M., Waters, S. J., & Keefe, F. J. (2003). Anger and persistent pain: Current status and future directions. *Pain, 103,* 1-5.

Janssen, S. A., Spinhoven, P., & Brosschot, J. F. (2001). Experimentally induced anger, cardiovascular reactivity, and pain sensitivity. *Journal of Psychosomatic Research, 51,* 479-485.

Materazzo, F., Cathcart, S., & Pritchard, D. (2000). Anger, depression, and coping interactions in headache activity and adjustment: A controlled study. *Journal of Psychosomatic Research, 49,* 69-75.

Anterior cingulate

Casey, K. L., & Bushnell, M. C. (2000). *Pain imaging.* Seattle: IASP Press.

Franken, I. H. (2003). Drug craving and addiction: Integrating psychological and neuropsychopharmacological approaches. *Progress in Neuro-Psychopharmacology and Biological Psychiatry, 27,* 563-579.

Hart, R. P., Wade, J. B., & Martelli, M. F. (2003). Cognitive impairment in patients with chronic pain: The significance of stress. *Current Pain and Headache Reports, 7,* 116-126.

Nutt, D., Lingford-Hughes, A., & Daglish, M. (2003). Future directions in substance dependence research. *Journal of Neural Transmission Supplement,* 95-103.

Peyron, R., Laurent, B., & Garcia-Larrea, L. (2000). Functional imaging of brain responses to pain: A review and meta-analysis. *Clinical Neurophysiology, 30,* 263-288.

Phillips, M. L., Drevets, W. C., Rauch, S. L., & Lane, R. (2003). Neurobiology of emotion perception II: Implications for major psychiatric disorders. *Biological Psychiatry, 54,* 515-528.

Rainville, P. (2002). Brain mechanisms of pain affect and pain modulation. *Current Opinion in Neurobiology, 12,* 195-204.

Rainville, P., Duncan, G. H., Price, D. D., Carrier, B., & Bushnell, M. C. (1997). Pain affect encoded in human anterior cingulate but not somatosensory cortex. *Science, 277,* 968-971.

Rauch, S. L. (2003). Neuroimaging and neurocircuitry models pertaining to the neurosurgical treatment of psychiatric disorders. *Neurosurgery Clinics of America, 14,* 213-223.

Antidepressants

Coquoz, D., Porchet, H. C., & Dayer, P. (1993). Central analgesic effects of desipramine, fluvoxamine, and moclobemide after single oral dosing: A study in healthy volunteers. *Clinical Pharmacology & Therapeutics, 54,* 339-344.

Enggaard, T. P., Klitgaard, N. A., Gram, L. F., Arendt-Nielsen, L., & Sindrup, S. H. (2001). Specific effect of venlafaxine on single and repetitive experimental painful stimuli in humans. *Clinical Pharmacology & Therapeutics, 69,* 245-251.

Enggaard, T. P., Poulsen, L., Arendt-Nielsen, L., Hansen, S. H., Bjornsdottir, I., Gram, L. F., & Sindrup, S. H. (2001). The analgesic effect of codeine as compared to imipramine in different human experimental pain models. *Pain, 92,* 277-282.

Fishbain, D. A., Cutler, R. B., Rosomoff, H. L., & Rosomoff, R. S. (1998). Do antidepressants have an analgesic effect in psychogenic pain and somatoform pain disorder? A meta-analysis. *Psychosomatic Medicine, 60,* 503-509.

Jackson, J. L., O'Malley, P. G., Tomkins, G., Balden, E., Santoro, J., & Kroenke, K. (2000). Treatment of functional gastrointestinal disorders with antidepressant medications: A meta-analysis. *The American Journal of Medicine, 108,* 65-72.

McQuay, H. J. (2002). Neuropathic pain: Evidence matters. *European Journal of Pain, Supplement 6,* 11-18.

McQuay, H. J., Tramer, M., Nye, B. A., Carroll, D., Wiffen, P. J., & Moore, R. A. (1996). A systematic review of antidepressants in neuropathic pain. *Pain, 68,* 217-227.

O'Malley, P. G., Balden, E., Tomkins, G., Santoro, J., Kroenke, K., & Jackson, J. L. (2000). Treatment of fibromyalgia with antidepressants: a meta-analysis. *Journal of General Internal Medicine, 15,* 659-666.

Onghena, P., & Van Houdenhove, B. (1992). Antidepressant-induced analgesia in chronic non-malignant pain: A meta-analysis of 39 placebo-controlled studies. *Pain, 49,* 205-219.

Peghini, P. L., Katz, P. O., & Castell, D. O. (1998). Imipramine decreases oesophageal pain perception in human male volunteers. *Gut, 42,* 807-813.

Rao, S. G. (2002). The neuropharmacology of centrally-acting analgesic medications in fibromyalgia. *Rheumatic Diseases Clinics of North America, 28,* 235-259.

Salerno, S. M., Browning, R., & Jackson, J. L. (2002). The effect of antidepressant treatment on chronic back pain: A meta-analysis. *Archives of Internal Medicine, 162,* 19-24.

Tomkins, G. E., Jackson, J. L., O'Malley, P. G., Balden, E., & Santoro, J. E. (2001). Treatment of chronic headache with antidepressants: A meta-analysis. *The American Journal of Medicine, 111,* 54-63.

Wallace, M. S., Barger, D., & Schulteis, G. (2002). The effect of chronic oral desipramine on capsaicin-induced allodynia and hyperalgesia: A double-blinded, placebo-controlled, crossover study. *Anesthesia Analgesia, 95,* 973-978.

Anxiety

Croog, S. H., Baume, R. M., & Nalbandian, J. (1995). Pre-surgery psychological characteristics, pain response, and activities impairment in female patients with repeated periodontal surgery. *Journal of Psychosomatic Research, 39,* 39-51.

Edwards, R. R., Augustson, E., & Fillingim, R. B. (2000). Sex-specific effects of pain-related anxiety on adjustment to chronic pain. *Clinical Journal of Pain, 16,* 46-53.

Edwards, R. R., Augustson, E., & Fillingim, R. B. (2003). Differential relationships between anxiety and treatment-associated pain reduction among male and female chronic pain patients. *Clinical Journal of Pain, 19,* 208-216.

Fillingim, R. B., Keefe, F. J., Light, K. C., Booker, D. K., & Maixner, W. (1996). The influence of gender and psychological factors on pain perception. *Journal of Gender, Culture, and Health, 1,* 21-36.

Fillingim, R. B., Maixner, W., Kincaid, S., Sigurdsson, A., & Harris, M. B. (1996). Pain sensitivity in patients with temporomandibular disorders: Relationship to clinical and psychosocial factors. *Clinical Journal of Pain, 12,* 260-269.

Gil, K. M., Ginsberg, B., Muir, M., Sykes, D., & Williams, D. A. (1990). Patient-controlled analgesia in postoperative pain: The relation of psychological factors to pain and analgesic use. *Clinical Journal of Pain, 2,* 137-142.

Graffenried, B. V., Adler, R., Abt, K., Nuesch, E., & Spiegel, R. (1978). The influence of anxiety and pain sensitivity on experimental pain in man. *Pain, 4,* 253-263.

Jones, A., Zachariae, R., & Arendt-Nielsen, L. (2003). Dispositional anxiety and the experience of pain: Gender-specific effects. *European Journal of Pain, 7,* 387-395.

Kain, Z. N., Sevarino, F., Alexander, G. M., Pincus, S., & Mayes, L. C. (2000). Preoperative anxiety and postoperative pain in women undergoing hysterectomy. A repeated-measures design. *Journal of Psychosomatic Research, 49,* 417-422.

McCracken, L. M., & Gross, R. T. (1993). Does anxiety affect coping with chronic pain? *Clinical Journal of Pain, 9,* 253-259.

McCracken, L. M., Gross, R. T., Aikens, J., & Carnrike, C. L., Jr. (1996). The assessment of anxiety and fear in persons with chronic pain: A comparison of instruments. *Behaviour Research and Therapy, 34,* 927-933.

McCracken, L. M., Gross, R. T., & Eccleston, C. (2002). Multimethod assessment of treatment process in chronic low back pain: Comparison of reported pain-related anxiety with directly measured physical capacity. *Behaviour Research and Therapy, 40,* 585-594.

McCracken, L. M., & Houle, T. (2000). Sex-specific and general roles of pain-related anxiety in adjustment to chronic pain: A reply to Edwards et al. *Clinical Journal of Pain, 16,* 275-276.

McCracken, L. M., Spertus, I. L., Janeck, A. S., Sinclair, D., & Wetzel, F. T. (1999). Behavioral dimensions of adjustment in persons with chronic pain: Pain-related anxiety and acceptance. *Pain, 80,* 283-289.

McWilliams, L. A., Cox, B. J., & Enns, M. W. (2003). Mood and anxiety disorders associated with chronic pain: An examination in a nationally representative sample. *Pain, 106,* 127-133.

Nelson, F. V., Zimmerman, L., Barnason, S., Nieveen, J., & Schmaderer, M. (1998). The relationship and influence of anxiety on postoperative pain in the coronary artery bypass graft patient. *Journal of Pain and Symptom Management, 15,* 102-109.

Perry, F., Parker, R. K., White, P. F., & Clifford, P. A. (1994). Role of psychological factors in postoperative pain control and recovery with patient-controlled analgesia. *Clinical Journal of Pain, 10,* 57-63.

Rhudy, J. L., & Meagher, M. W. (2000). Fear and anxiety: Divergent effects on human pain thresholds. *Pain, 84,* 65-75.

Riley, J. L., III, Robinson, M. E., Wade, J. B., Myers, C. D., & Price, D. D. (2001). Sex differences in negative emotional responses to chronic pain. *Journal of Pain, 2,* 354-359.

Robin, O., Vinard, H., Vernet Maury, E., & Saumet, J. L. (1987). Influence of sex and anxiety on pain threshold and tolerance. *Functional Neurology, 2,* 173-179.

Robinson, M. E., & Riley, J. L. I. (1999). The role of emotion in pain. In R. J. Gatchel & D. C. Turk (Eds.), *Psychosocial factors in pain* (pp. 74-88). New York: Guilford Press.

Anxiety sensitivity

Asmundson, G. J., Norton, P. J., & Norton, G. R. (1999). Beyond pain: The role of fear and avoidance in chronicity. *Clinical Psychology Review, 19,* 97-119.

Asmundson, G. J., Norton, P. J., & Veloso, F. (1999). Anxiety sensitivity and fear of pain in patients with recurring headaches. *Behaviour Research and Therapy, 37,* 703-713.

Asmundson, G. J., Wright, K. D., Norton, P. J., & Veloso, F. (2001). Anxiety sensitivity and other emotionality traits in predicting headache medication use in patients with recurring headaches: Implications for abuse and dependency. *Addictive Behavior, 26,* 827-840.

Keogh, E., & Chaloner, N. (2002). The moderating effect of anxiety sensitivity on caffeine-induced hypoalgesia in healthy women. *Psychopharmacology, 164,* 429-431.

Keogh, E., & Cochrane, M. (2002). Anxiety sensitivity, cognitive biases, and the experience of pain. *Journal of Pain, 3,* 320-329.

Keogh, E., & Mansoor, L. (2001). Investigating the effects of anxiety sensitivity and coping on the perception of cold pressor pain in healthy women. *European Journal of Pain, 5,* 11-22.

Muris, P., Vlaeyen, J., & Meesters, C. (2001). The relationship between anxiety sensitivity and fear of pain in healthy adolescents. *Behaviour Research and Therapy, 39,* 1357-1368.

Norton, G. R., Norton, P. J., Asmundson, G. J., Thompson, L. A., & Larsen, D. K. (1999). Neurotic butterflies in my stomach: The role of anxiety, anxiety sensitivity and depression in functional gastrointestinal disorders. *Journal of Psychosomatic Research, 47,* 233-240.

Reiss, S., Peterson, R. A., Gursky, D. M., & McNally, R. J. (1986). Anxiety sensitivity, anxiety frequency and the prediction of fearfulness. *Behaviour Research and Therapy, 24,* 1-8.

Beck Depression Inventory

Beck, A. T., Stees, R. A., & Garbin, M. G. (1988). Psychometric properties of the Beck Depression Inventory: Twenty-five years of evaluation. *Clinical Psychology Reviews, 8,* 77-100.

Dworkin, S. F., Sherman, J., Mancl, L., Ohrbach, R., LeResche, L., & Truelove, E. (2002). Reliability, validity, and clinical utility of the research diagnostic criteria for Temporomandibular Disorders Axis II Scales: Depression, non-specific physical symptoms, and graded chronic pain. *Journal of Orofacial Pain, 16,* 207-220.

Geisser, M. E., Roth, R. S., & Robinson, M. E. (1997). Assessing depression among persons with chronic pain using the Center for Epidemiological Studies-Depression Scale and the Beck Depression Inventory: A comparative analysis. *Clinical Journal of Pain, 13,* 163-170.

Holzberg, A. D., Robinson, M. E., Geisser, M. E., & Gremillion, H. A. (1996). The effects of depression and chronic pain on psychosocial and physical functioning. *Clinical Journal of Pain, 12,* 118-125.

Lebovits, A. H. (2000). The psychological assessment of patients with chronic pain. *Current Review of Pain, 4,* 122-126.

Morley, S., Williams, A. C., & Black, S. (2002). A confirmatory factor analysis of the Beck Depression Inventory in chronic pain. *Pain, 99,* 289-298.

Skevington, S. M., Carse, M. S., & Williams, A. C. (2001). Validation of the WHOQOL-100: Pain management improves quality of life for chronic pain patients. *Clinical Journal of Pain, 17,* 264-275.

Wesley, A. L., Gatchel, R. J., Garofalo, J. P., & Polatin, P. B. (1999). Toward more accurate use of the Beck Depression Inventory with chronic back pain patients. *Clinical Journal of Pain, 15,* 117-121.

Williams, A. C., & Richardson, P. H. (1993). What does the BDI measure in chronic pain? *Pain, 55,* 259-266.

Behavioral factors

Flor, H., Birbaumer, N., Schulz, R., Grusser, S. M., & Mucha, R. F. (2002). Pavlovian conditioning of opioid and nonopioid pain inhibitory mechanisms in humans. *European Journal of Pain, 6,* 395-402.

Flor, H., Knost, B., & Birbaumer, N. (2002). The role of operant conditioning in chronic pain: An experimental investigation. *Pain, 95,* 111-118.

Fordyce, W. E. (1976). *Behavioral methods for chronic pain and illness.* St. Louis: Mosby.

Guck, T. P., Skultety, F. M., Meilman, P. W., & Dowd, E. T. (1985). Multidisciplinary pain center follow-up study: Evaluation with a no-treatment control group. *Pain, 21,* 295-306.

Keefe, F. J., Crisson, J. E., Maltbie, A., Bradley, L., & Gil, K. M. (1986). Illness behavior as a predictor of pain and overt behavior patterns in chronic low back pain patients. *Journal of Psychosomatic Research, 30,* 543-551.

Keefe, F. J., & Dolan, E. (1986). Pain behavior and pain coping strategies in low back pain and myofascial pain dysfunction syndrome patients. *Pain, 24,* 49-56.

Keefe, F. J., & Hill, R. W. (1985). An objective approach to quantifying pain behavior and gait patterns in low back pain patients. *Pain, 21,* 153-161.

Keefe, F. J., Wilkins, R. H., & Cook, W. A. (1984). Direct observation of pain behavior in low back pain patients during physical examination. *Pain, 20,* 59-68.

Roberts, A. H., & Reinhardt, L. (1980). The behavioral management of chronic pain: long-term follow-up with comparison groups. *Pain, 8,* 151-162.

Vlaeyen, J. W., de Jong, J., Geilen, M., Heuts, P. H., & van Breukelen, G. (2002). The treatment of fear of movement/(re)injury in chronic low back pain: Further evidence on the effectiveness of exposure in vivo. *Clinical Journal of Pain, 18,* 251-261.

Beliefs

DeGood, D. E., & Tait, R. C. (2001). Assessment of pain beliefs and pain coping. In D. C. Turk & R. Melzack (Eds.), *Handbook of pain assessment* (pp. 320-345). New York: Guilford Press.

Herda, C. A., Siegeris, K., & Basler, H. D. (1994). The Pain Beliefs and Perceptions Inventory: Further evidence for a 4-factor structure. *Pain, 57,* 85-90.

Jensen, M. P., & Karoly, P. (1992). Pain-specific beliefs, perceived symptom severity, and adjustment to chronic pain. *Clinical Journal of Pain, 8,* 123-130.

Jensen, M. P., Karoly, P., & Huger, R. (1987). The development and preliminary validation of an instrument to assess patients' attitudes toward pain. *Journal of Psychosomatic Research, 31,* 393-400.

Jensen, M. P., Romano, J. M., Turner, J. A., Good, A. B., & Wald, L. H. (1999). Patient beliefs predict patient functioning: Further support for a cognitive-behavioural model of chronic pain. *Pain, 81,* 95-104.

Jensen, M. P., Turner, J. A., & Romano, J. M. (2000). Pain belief assessment: A comparison of short and long versions of the Survey of Pain Attitudes. *Journal of Pain, 1,* 138-150.

Jensen, M. P., Turner, J. A., & Romano, J. M. (2001). Changes in beliefs, catastrophizing, and coping are associated with improvement in multidisciplinary pain treatment. *Journal of Consulting and Clinical Psychology, 69,* 655-662.

Jensen, M. P., Turner, J. A., Romano, J. M., & Lawler, B. K. (1994). Relationship of pain-specific beliefs to chronic pain adjustment. *Pain, 57,* 301-309.

Morley, S., & Wilkinson, L. (1995). The Pain Beliefs and Perceptions Inventory: A British replication. *Pain, 61,* 427-433.

Tait, R. C., & Chibnall, J. T. (1997). Development of a brief version of the Survey of Pain Attitudes. *Pain, 70,* 229-235.

Tait, R. C., & Chibnall, J. T. (1998). Attitude profiles and clinical status in patients with chronic pain. *Pain, 78,* 49-57.

Williams, D. A., & Keefe, F. J. (1991). Pain beliefs and the use of cognitive-behavioral coping strategies. *Pain, 46,* 185-190.

Williams, D. A., Robinson, M. E., & Geisser, M. E. (1994). Pain beliefs: Assessment and utility. *Pain, 59,* 71-78.

Williams, D. A., & Thorn, B. E. (1989). An empirical assessment of pain beliefs. *Pain, 36,* 351-358.

Biofeedback

Bush, C., Ditto, B., & Feuerstein, M. (1985). A controlled evaluation of paraspinal EMG biofeedback in the treatment of chronic low back pain. *Health Psychology, 4,* 307-321.

Holroyd, K. A., Penzien, D. B., Hursey, K. G., Tobin, D. L., Rogers, L., Holm, J. E., Marcille, P. J., Hall, J. R., & Chila, A. G. (1984). Change mechanisms in EMG biofeedback training: Cognitive changes underlying improvements in tension headache. *Journal of Consulting and Clinical Psychology, 52,* 1039-1053.

Myers, C. D., White, B. A., & Heft, M. W. (2002). A review of complementary and alternative medicine use for treating chronic facial pain. *Journal of the American Dental Association, 133,* 1189-1196.

Newton-John, T. R., Spence, S. H., & Schotte, D. (1995). Cognitive-behavioural therapy versus EMG biofeedback in the treatment of chronic low back pain. *Behaviour Research and Therapy, 33,* 691-697.

Nielson, W. R., & Weir, R. (2001). Biopsychosocial approaches to the treatment of chronic pain. *Clinical Journal of Pain, 17,* S114-S127.

Turk, D. C., Zaki, H. S., & Rudy, T. E. (1993). Effects of intraoral appliance and biofeedback/stress management alone and in combination in treating pain and depression in patients with temporomandibular disorders. *The Journal of Prosthetic Dentistry, 70,* 158-164.

Biopsychosocial model

Turk, D. C. (1996). Biopsychosocial perspective on chronic pain. In R. J. Gatchel & D. C. Turk (Eds.), *Psychological approaches to pain management: A practitioner's handbook* (pp. 3-32). New York: Guilford Press.

Cancer pain

Anderson, K. O., Syrjala, K. L., & Cleeland, C. S. (2001). How to assess cancer pain. In D. C. Turk & R. Melzack (Eds.), *Handbook of pain assessment* (2nd ed., pp. 579-598). New York: The Guilford Press.

Breitbart, W. S., & Payne, D. K. (2004). Psychological and psychiatric dimensions of palliative care. In R. H. Dworkin & W. S. Breitbart (Eds.), *Psychosocial aspects of pain: A handbook for health care providers* (pp. 427-461). Seattle: IASP Press.

Cleeland, C. S., Gonin, R., Hatfield, A. K., Edmonson, J. H., Blum, R. H., Stewart, J. A., & Pandya, K. J. (1994). Pain and its treatment in outpatients with metastatic cancer. *New England Journal of Medicine, 330,* 592-596.

Devine, E. C. (2003). Meta-analysis of the effect of psychoeducational interventions on pain in adults with cancer. *Oncology Nursing Forum, 30,* 75-89.

Fortner, B. V., Okon, T. A., & Portenoy, R. K. (2002). A survey of pain-related hospitalizations, emergency department visits, and physician office visits reported by cancer patients with and without history of breakthrough pain. *Journal of Pain, 3,* 38-44.

Herndon, J. E., Fleishman, S., Kornblith, A. B., Kosty, M., Green, M. R., & Holland, J. (1999). Is quality of life predictive of the survival of patients with advanced nonsmall cell lung carcinoma? *Cancer, 85,* 333-340.

Page, G. G., Blakely, W. P., & Ben Eliyahu, S. (2001). Evidence that postoperative pain is a mediator of the tumor-promoting effects of surgery in rats. *Pain, 90,* 191-199.

Portenoy, R. K., Thaler, H. T., Kornblith, A. B., Lepore, J. M., Friedlander-Klar, H., Coyle, N., Smart-Curley, T., Kemeny, N., Norton, L., & Hoskins, W. (1994). Symptom prevalence, characteristics and distress in a cancer population. *Quality of Life Research, 3,* 183-189.

World Health Organization (1996). *Cancer pain relief: With a guide to opioid availability.* Geneva: WHO.

Zaza, C., & Baine, N. (2002). Cancer pain and psychosocial factors: A critical review of the literature. *Journal of Pain and Symptom Management, 24,* 526-542.

Catastrophizing

Burns, J. W., Kubilus, A., Bruehl, S., Harden, R. N., & Lofland, K. (2003). Do changes in cognitive factors influence outcome following multidisciplinary treatment for chronic pain? A cross-lagged panel analysis. *Journal of Consulting and Clinical Psychology, 71,* 81-91.

Campbell, C. M., Edwards, R. R., & Fillingim, R. B. (2005). Ethnic differences in responses to multiple experimental pain stimuli. *Pain, 113,* 20-26.

Fillingim, R. B., Wilkinson, C. S., & Powell, T. (1999). Self-reported abuse history and pain complaints among healthy young adults. *Clinical Journal of Pain, 15,* 85-91.

France, C. R., France, J. L., al'Absi, M., Ring, C., & McIntyre, D. (2002). Catastrophizing is related to pain ratings, but not nociceptive flexion reflex threshold. *Pain, 99,* 459-463.

Geisser, M. E., Robinson, M. E., & Pickren, W. E. (1992). Differences in cognitive coping strategies among pain-sensitive and pain-tolerant individuals on the cold pressor test. *Behavior Therapy, 23,* 31-42.

Keefe, F. J., Lefebvre, J. C., Egert, J. R., Affleck, G., Sullivan, M. J., & Caldwell, D. S. (2000). The relationship of gender to pain, pain behavior, and disability in osteoarthritis patients: The role of catastrophizing. *Pain, 87,* 325-334.

Osman, A., Barrios, F. X., Gutierrez, P. M., Kopper, B. A., Merrifield, T., & Grittmann, L. (2000). The Pain Catastrophizing Scale: Further psychometric evaluation with adult samples. *Journal of Behavioral Medicine, 23,* 351-365.

Rosenstiel, A. K., & Keefe, F. J. (1983). The use of coping strategies in chronic low back pain patients: Relationship to patient characteristics and current adjustment. *Pain, 17,* 33-44.

Sullivan, M. J., Bishop, S., & Pivik, J. (1995). The Pain Catastrophizing Scale: Development and validation. *Psychological Assessment, 7,* 524-532.

Sullivan, M. J., Thorn, B., Haythornthwaite, J. A., Keefe, F., Martin, M., Bradley, L. A., & Lefebvre, J. C. (2001). Theoretical perspectives on the relation between catastrophizing and pain. *Clinical Journal of Pain, 17,* 52-64.

Thorn, B. E., Ward, L. C., Sullivan, M. J., & Boothby, J. L. (2003). Communal coping model of catastrophizing: Conceptual model building. *Pain, 106,* 1-2.

Chest pain

Bradley, L. A., Richter, J. E., Scarinci, I. C., Haile, J. M., & Schan, C. A. (1992). Psychosocial and psychophysical assessments of patients with unexplained chest pain. *American Journal of Medicine, 92,* 65S-73S.

Brorsson, B., Bernstein, S. J., Brook, R. H., & Werko, L. (2002). Quality of life of patients with chronic stable angina before and four years after coronary revascularisation compared with a normal population. *Heart, 87,* 140-145.

Eslick, G. D., Jones, M. P., & Talley, N. J. (2003). Non-cardiac chest pain: Prevalence, risk factors, impact and consulting—A population-based study. *Alimentary Pharmacology & Therapeutics, 17,* 1115-1124.

Kiebzak, G. M., Pierson, L. M., Campbell, M., & Cook, J. W. (2002). Use of the SF36 general health status survey to document health-related quality of life in patients with coronary artery disease: Effect of disease and response to coronary artery bypass graft surgery. *Heart & Lung, 31,* 207-213.

Kroenke, K., Arrington, M. E., & Mangelsdorff, A. D. (1990). The prevalence of symptoms in medical outpatients and the adequacy of therapy. *Archives of Internal Medicine, 150,* 1685-1689.

Lewin, B. (1997). The psychological and behavioral management of angina. *Journal of Psychosomatic Research, 43,* 453-462.

Lewin, R. J., Furze, G., Robinson, J., Griffith, K., Wiseman, S., Pye, M., & Boyle, R. (2002). A randomised controlled trial of a self-management plan for patients with newly diagnosed angina. *British Journal of General Practice, 52,* 194-196.

Miller, P. F., Light, K. C., Bragdon, E. E., Ballenger, M. N., Herbst, M. C., Maixner, W., Hinderliter, A. L., Atkinson, S. S., Koch, G. G., & Sheps, D. S. (1993). Beta-endorphin response to exercise and mental stress in patients with ischemic heart disease. *Journal of Psychosomatic Research, 37,* 455-465.

Rumsfeld, J. S., Magid, D. J., Plomondon, M. E., Sales, A. E., Grunwald, G. K., Every, N. R., & Spertus, J. A. (2003). History of depression, angina, and quality of life after acute coronary syndromes. *American Heart Journal, 145,* 493-499.

Spertus, J. A., Dewhurst, T. A., Dougherty, C. M., Nichol, P., McDonell, M., Bliven, B., & Fihn, S. D. (2002). Benefits of an "angina clinic" for patients with coronary artery disease: A demonstration of health status measures as markers of health care quality. *American Heart Journal, 143,* 145-150.

Thurston, R. C., Keefe, F. J., Bradley, L., Rama Krishnan, K. R., & Caldwell, D. S. (2001). Chest pain in the absence of coronary artery disease: A biopsychosocial perspective. *Pain, 93,* 95-100.

Children

Anand, K. J. (2001). Consensus statement for the prevention and management of pain in the newborn. *Archives of Pediatrics & Adolescent Medicine, 155,* 173-180.

Anthony, K. K., & Schanberg, L. E. (2001). Juvenile primary fibromyalgia syndrome. *Current Rheumatology Reports, 3,* 165-171.

Eccleston, C., Morley, S., Williams, A., Yorke, L., & Mastroyannopoulou, K. (2002). Systematic review of randomised controlled trials of psychological therapy for chronic pain in children and adolescents, with a subset meta-analysis of pain relief. *Pain, 99,* 157-165.

Hunfeld, J. A., Perquin, C. W., Bertina, W., Hazebroek-Kampschreur, A. A., Suijlekom-Smit, L. W., Koes, B. W., van der Wouden, J. C., & Passchier, J. (2002). Stability of pain parameters and pain-related quality of life in adolescents with persistent pain: A three-year follow-up. *Clinical Journal of Pain, 18,* 99-106.

Hunfeld, J. A., Perquin, C. W., Duivenvoorden, H. J., Hazebroek-Kampschreur, A. A., Passchier, J., Suijlekom-Smit, L. W., & van der Wouden, J. C. (2001). Chronic pain and its impact on quality of life in adolescents and their families. *Journal of Pediatric Psychology, 26,* 145-153.

Kashikar-Zuck, S., Goldschneider, K. R., Powers, S. W., Vaught, M. H., & Hershey, A. D. (2001). Depression and functional disability in chronic pediatric pain. *Clinical Journal of Pain, 17,* 341-349.

Malleson, P., & Clinch, J. (2003). Pain syndromes in children. *Current Opinion in Rheumatology, 15,* 572-580.

McGrath, P. A., & Gillespie, J. (2001). Pain assessment in children and adolescents. In D. C. Turk & R. Melzack (Eds.), *Handbook of pain assessment* (pp. 97-118). New York: Guilford Press.

McGrath, P. A., Speechley, K. N., Seifert, C. E., Biehn, J. T., Cairney, A. E., Gorodzinsky, F. P., Dickie, G. L., McCusker, P. J., & Morrissy, J. R. (2000). A survey of children's acute, recurrent, and chronic pain: Validation of the pain experience interview. *Pain, 87,* 59-73.

McGrath, P. J., & Finley, G. A. (2003). *Pediatric pain: Biological and social context.* Seattle: IASP Press.

Merlijn, V. P., Hunfeld, J. A., van der Wouden, J. C., Hazebroek-Kampschreur, A. A., Koes, B. W., & Passchier, J. (2003). Psychosocial factors associated with chronic pain in adolescents. *Pain, 101,* 33-43.

Morison, S. J., Grunau, R. E., Oberlander, T. F., & Whitfield, M. F. (2001). Relations between behavioral and cardiac autonomic reactivity to acute pain in preterm neonates. *Clinical Journal of Pain, 17,* 350-358.

Morison, S. J., Holsti, L., Grunau, R. E., Whitfield, M. F., Oberlander, T. F., Chan, H. W., & Williams, L. (2003). Are there developmentally distinct motor indicators of pain in preterm infants? *Early Human Development, 72,* 131-146.

Palermo, T. M. (2000). Impact of recurrent and chronic pain on child and family daily functioning: A critical review of the literature. *Journal of Developmental & Behavioral Pediatrics, 21,* 58-69.

Porter, F. L., Grunau, R. E., & Anand, K. J. (1999). Long-term effects of pain in infants. *Journal of Developmental & Behavioral Pediatrics, 20,* 253-261.

Powers, S. W. (1999). Empirically supported treatments in pediatric psychology: Procedure-related pain. *Journal of Pediatric Psychology, 24,* 131-145.

Ruda, M. A., Ling, Q. D., Hohmann, A. G., Peng, Y. B., & Tachibana, T. (2000). Altered nociceptive neuronal circuits after neonatal peripheral inflammation. *Science, 289,* 628-631.

Schanberg, L. E., Anthony, K. K., Gil, K. M., Lefebvre, J. C., Kredich, D. W., & Macharoni, L. M. (2001). Family pain history predicts child health status in children with chronic rheumatic disease. *Pediatrics, 108,* E47.

Weydert, J. A., Ball, T. M., & Davis, M. F. (2003). Systematic review of treatments for recurrent abdominal pain. *Pediatrics, 111,* e1-e11.

Chronic pain

Gallagher, R. M. (1999). Primary care and pain medicine. A community solution to the public health problem of chronic pain. *Medical Clinics of North America, 83,* v, 555-583.

Cognitive-behavioral therapy

Burns, J. W., Kubilus, A., Bruehl, S., Harden, R. N., & Lofland, K. (2003). Do changes in cognitive factors influence outcome following multidisciplinary treatment for chronic pain? A cross-lagged panel analysis. *Journal of Consulting and Clinical Psychology, 71,* 81-91.

Eccleston, C., Morley, S., Williams, A., Yorke, L., & Mastroyannopoulou, K. (2002). Systematic review of randomised controlled trials of psychological therapy for chronic pain in children and adolescents, with a subset meta-analysis of pain relief. *Pain, 99,* 157-165.

Jensen, M. P., Turner, J. A., & Romano, J. M. (1994). Correlates of improvement in multidisciplinary treatment of chronic pain. *Journal of Consulting and Clinical Psychology, 62,* 172-179.

Jensen, M. P., Turner, J. A., & Romano, J. M. (2001). Changes in beliefs, catastrophizing, and coping are associated with improvement in multidisciplinary pain treatment. *Journal of Consulting and Clinical Psychology, 69,* 655-662.

Morley, S., Eccleston, C., & Williams, A. (1999). Systematic review and meta-analysis of randomized controlled trials of cognitive behaviour therapy and behaviour therapy for chronic pain in adults, excluding headache. *Pain, 80,* 1-13.

Turk, D. C., & Rudy, T. E. (1989). A cognitive-behavioral perspective on chronic pain: Beyond the scalpel and the syringe. In C. D. Tollison (Ed.), *Handbook of chronic pain management* (pp. 222-236). Baltimore: Williams & Wilkins.

van Tulder, M. W., Ostelo, R., Vlaeyen, J. W., Linton, S. J., Morley, S. J., & Assendelft, W. J. (2001). Behavioral treatment for chronic low back pain: A systematic review within the framework of the Cochrane Back Review Group. *Spine, 26,* 270-281.

Complex regional pain syndrome

Bennett, G. J., & Harden, R. N. (2003). Questions concerning the incidence and prevalence of complex regional pain syndrome type I (RSD). *Pain, 106,* 209-210.

Bruehl, S., Chung, O. Y., & Burns, J. W. (2003). Differential effects of expressive anger regulation on chronic pain intensity in CRPS and non-CRPS limb pain patients. *Pain, 104,* 647-654.

Bruehl, S., Husfeldt, B., Lubenow, T. R., Nath, H., & Ivankovich, A. D. (1996). Psychological differences between reflex sympathetic dystrophy and non-RSD chronic pain patients. *Pain, 67,* 107-114.

Feldman, S. I., Downey, G., & Schaffer-Neitz, R. (1999). Pain, negative mood, and perceived support in chronic pain patients: A daily diary study of people with reflex sympathetic dystrophy syndrome. *Journal of Consulting and Clinical Psychology, 67,* 776-785.

Geertzen, J. H., Bruijn-Kofman, A. T., de Bruijn, H. P., van de Wiel, H. B., & Dijkstra, P. U. (1998). Stressful life events and psychological dysfunction in Complex Regional Pain Syndrome type I. *Clinical Journal of Pain, 14,* 143-147.

Geertzen, J. H., Dijkstra, P. U., Groothoff, J. W., ten Duis, H. J., & Eisma, W. H. (1998). Reflex sympathetic dystrophy of the upper extremity—A 5.5-year follow-up. Part II. Social life events, general health and changes in occupation. *Acta Orthopaedica Scandinavica Supplement, 279,* 19-23.

Kemler, M. A., Schouten, H. J., & Gracely, R. H. (2000). Diagnosing sensory abnormalities with either normal values or values from contralateral skin: Comparison of two approaches in complex regional pain syndrome I. *Anesthesiology, 93,* 718-727.

Merskey, H., & Bogduk, N. (1994). *Classification of chronic pain* (2nd ed.). Seattle: IASP Press.

Rommel, O., Malin, J., Zenz, M., & Janig, W. (2001). Quantitative sensory testing, neurophysiological and psychological examination in patients with complex regional pain syndrome and hemisensory deficits. *Pain, 93,* 279-293.

Sandroni, P., Benrud-Larson, L. M., McClelland, R. L., & Low, P. A. (2003). Complex regional pain syndrome type I: Incidence and prevalence in Olmsted county, a population-based study. *Pain, 103,* 199-207.

Consciousness

Chapman, C. R. (1999). Chronic pain and consicousness: A constructivist perspective. In R. J. Gatchel & D. C. Turk (Eds.), *Psychosocial factors in pain* (pp. 35-55). New York: Guilford Press.

Conversion disorder

American Psychiatric Association (1994). *Diagnostic and statistical manual of mental disorders: DSM-IV* (4th ed.). Washington, DC: American Psychiatric Association.

Coping

Bandura, A., O'Leary, A., Taylor, C. B., Gauthier, J., & Gossard, D. (1987). Perceived self-efficacy and pain control: Opioid and nonopioid mechanisms. *Journal of Personality and Social Psychology, 53,* 563-571.

Brown, G. K., & Nicassio, P. M. (1987). Development of a questionnaire for the assessment of active and passive coping strategies in chronic pain patients. *Pain, 31,* 53-64.

Burns, J. W., Kubilus, A., Bruehl, S., Harden, R. N., & Lofland, K. (2003). Do changes in cognitive factors influence outcome following multidisciplinary treatment for chronic pain? A cross-lagged panel analysis. *Journal of Consulting and Clinical Psychology, 71,* 81-91.

France, C. R., France, J. L., al'Absi, M., Ring, C., & McIntyre, D. (2002). Catastrophizing is related to pain ratings, but not nociceptive flexion reflex threshold. *Pain, 99,* 459-463.

Geisser, M. E., Robinson, M. E., & Pickren, W. E. (1992). Differences in cognitive coping strategies among pain-sensitive and pain-tolerant individuals on the cold pressor test. *Behavior Therapy, 23,* 31-42.

Jacobsen, P. B., & Butler, R. W. (1996). Relation of cognitive coping and catastrophizing to acute pain and analgesic use following breast cancer surgery. *Journal of Behavioral Medicine, 19,* 17-29.

Jensen, M. P., Turner, J. A., & Romano, J. M. (1994). Correlates of improvement in multidisciplinary treatment of chronic pain. *Journal of Consulting and Clinical Psychology, 62,* 172-179.

Jensen, M. P., Turner, J. A., & Romano, J. M. (2001). Changes in beliefs, catastrophizing, and coping are associated with improvement in multidisciplinary pain treatment. *Journal of Consulting and Clinical Psychology, 69,* 655-662.

Jensen, M. P., Turner, J. A., Romano, J. M., & Karoly, P. (1991). Coping with chronic pain: A critical review of the literature. *Pain, 47,* 249-283.

Jensen, M. P., Turner, J. A., Romano, J. M., & Strom, S. E. (1995). The Chronic Pain Coping Inventory: Development and preliminary validation. *Pain, 60,* 203-216.

Lester, N., Lefebvre, J. C., & Keefe, F. J. (1996). Pain in young adults—III: Relationships of three pain-coping measures to pain and activity interference. *Clinical Journal of Pain, 12,* 291-300.

Nicassio, P. M., Schoenfeld-Smith, K., Radojevic, V., & Schuman, C. (1995). Pain coping mechanisms in fibromyalgia: Relationship to pain and functional outcomes. *Journal of Rheumatology, 22,* 1552-1558.

Riley, J. L., III, Robinson, M. E., & Geisser, M. E. (1999). Empirical subgroups of the Coping Strategies Questionnaire-Revised: A multisample study. *Clinical Journal of Pain, 15,* 111-116.

Robinson, M. E., Riley, J. L., III, Myers, C. D., Sadler, I. J., Kvaal, S. A., Geisser, M. E., & Keefe, F. J. (1997). The Coping Strategies Questionnaire: A large sample, item level factor analysis. *Clinical Journal of Pain, 13,* 43-49.

Rosenstiel, A. K., & Keefe, F. J. (1983). The use of coping strategies in chronic low back pain patients: Relationship to patient characteristics and current adjustment. *Pain, 17,* 33-44.

Swartzman, L. C., Gwadry, F. G., Shapiro, A. P., & Teasell, R. W. (1994). The factor structure of the Coping Strategies Questionnaire. *Pain, 57,* 311-316.

Tota-Faucette, M. E., Gil, K. M., Williams, D. A., Keefe, F. J., & Goli, V. (1993). Predictors of response to pain management treatment: The role of family environment and changes in cognitive processes. *Clinical Journal of Pain, 9,* 115-123.

Tripp, D. A., Stanish, W. D., Reardon, G., Coady, C., & Sullivan, M. J. (2003). Comparing postoperative pain experiences of the adolescent and adult athlete after anterior cruciate ligament surgery. *Journal of Athletic Training, 38,* 154-157.

Villemure, C., & Bushnell, M. C. (2002). Cognitive modulation of pain: How do attention and emotion influence pain processing? *Pain, 95,* 195-199.

Cortisol

al'Absi, M., Petersen, K. L., & Wittmers, L. E. (2002). Adrenocortical and hemodynamic predictors of pain perception in men and women. *Pain, 96,* 197-204.

Crofford, L. J. (1998). Neuroendocrine abnormalities in fibromyalgia and related disorders. *American Journal of the Medical Sciences, 315,* 359-366.

Greisen, J., Hokland, M., Grofte, T., Hansen, P. O., Jensen, T. S., Vilstrup, H., & Tonnesen, E. (1999). Acute pain induces an instant increase in natural killer cell cytotoxicity in humans and this response is abolished by local anaesthesia. *British Journal of Anaesthesia, 83,* 235-240.

Hurwitz, E. L., & Morgenstern, H. (2001). Immediate and long-term effects of immune stimulation: Hypothesis linking the immune response to subsequent physical and psychological wellbeing. *Medical Hypotheses, 56,* 620-624.

Jones, D. A., Rollman, G. B., & Brooke, R. I. (1997). The cortisol response to psychological stress in temporomandibular dysfunction. *Pain, 72,* 171-182.

Korszun, A., Young, E. A., Singer, K., Carlson, N. E., Brown, M. B., & Crofford, L. (2002). Basal circadian cortisol secretion in women with temporomandibular disorders. *Journal of Dental Research, 81,* 279-283.

Zimmer, C., Basler, H. D., Vedder, H., & Lautenbacher, S. (2003). Sex differences in cortisol response to noxious stress. *Clinical Journal of Pain, 19,* 233-239.

Depression

American Psychiatric Association (1994). *Diagnostic and statistical manual of mental disorders: DSM-IV* (4th ed.). Washington, DC: American Psychiatric Association.

Atkinson, J. H., Slater, M. A., Patterson, T. L., Grant, I., & Garfin, S. R. (1991). Prevalence, onset, and risk of psychiatric disorders in men with chronic low back pain: A controlled study. *Pain, 45,* 111-121.

Banks, S. M. & Kerns, R. D. (1996). Explaining high rates of depression in chronic pain: A diathesis-stress framework. *Psychological Bulletin, 119,* 95-110.

Bao, Y., Sturm, R., & Croghan, T. W. (2003). A national study of the effect of chronic pain on the use of health care by depressed persons. *Psychiatric Services, 54,* 693-697.

Beck, A. T., & Steer, R. A. (1987). *Beck depression inventory manual.* San Antonio, TX: Psychological Corporation.

Block, A. R. (1999). Presurgical psychological screening in chronic pain syndromes: Psychosocial risk factors for poor surgical results. In R. J. Gatchel & D. C. Turk (Eds.), *Psychosocial factors in pain* (pp. 390-411). New York: Guilford Press.

Blumer, D., & Heilbronn, M. (1982). Chronic pain as a variant of depressive disease: The pain-prone disorder. *Journal of Nervous and Mental Disease, 170,* 381-406.

Breslau, N., Lipton, R. B., Stewart, W. F., Schultz, L. R., & Welch, K. M. (2003). Comorbidity of migraine and depression: Investigating potential etiology and prognosis. *Neurology, 60,* 1308-1312.

Breslau, N., Schultz, L. R., Stewart, W. F., Lipton, R. B., Lucia, V. C., & Welch, K. M. (2000). Headache and major depression: is the association specific to migraine? *Neurology, 54,* 308-313.

Briley, M. (2003). New hope in the treatment of painful symptoms in depression. *Current Opinion in Investigational Drugs, 4,* 42-45.

Campbell, L. C., Clauw, D. J., & Keefe, F. J. (2003). Persistent pain and depression: A biopsychosocial perspective. *Biological Psychiatry, 54,* 399-409.

Dersh, J., Polatin, P. B., & Gatchel, R. J. (2002). Chronic pain and psychopathology: Research findings and theoretical considerations. *Psychosomatic Medicine, 64,* 773-786.

Egger, H. L., Costello, E. J., Erkanli, A., & Angold, A. (1999). Somatic complaints and psychopathology in children and adolescents: Stomach aches, musculoskeletal pains, and headaches. *Journal of the American Academy of Child & Adolescent Psychiatry, 38,* 852-860.

Fishbain, D. A., Cutler, R., Rosomoff, H. L., & Rosomoff, R. S. (1997). Chronic pain-associated depression: Antecedent or consequence of chronic pain? A review. *Clinical Journal of Pain, 13,* 116-137.

Gatchel, R. J. (1996). Psychological disorders and chronic pain: Cause-and-effect relationships. In R. J. Gatchel & D. C. Turk (Eds.), *Psychological approaches to pain management: A practitioner's handbook* (pp. 33-52). New York: Guilford Press.

Geisser, M. E., Roth, R. S., & Robinson, M. E. (1997). Assessing depression among persons with chronic pain using the Center for Epidemiological Studies—Depression Scale and the Beck Depression Inventory: A comparative analysis. *Clinical Journal of Pain, 13,* 163-170.

Greenberg, P. E., Leong, S. A., Birnbaum, H. G., & Robinson, R. L. (2003). The economic burden of depression with painful symptoms. *Journal of Clinical Psychiatry, 64* (Supplement 7), 17-23.

Haythornthwaite, J. A., Sieber, W. J., & Kerns, R. D. (1991). Depression and the chronic pain experience. *Pain, 46,* 177-184.

Holzberg, A. D., Robinson, M. E., Geisser, M. E., & Gremillion, H. A. (1996). The effects of depression and chronic pain on psychosocial and physical functioning. *Clinical Journal of Pain, 12,* 118-125.

Hotopf, M., Mayou, R., Wadsworth, M., & Wessely, S. (1998). Temporal relationships between physical symptoms and psychiatric disorder. Results from a national birth cohort. *British Journal of Psychiatry, 173,* 255-261.

Hudson, J. I., Goldenberg, D. L., Pope, H. G. J., Keck, P. E. J., & Schlesinger, L. (1992). Comorbidity of fibromyalgia with medical and psychiatric disorders. *American Journal of Medicine, 92,* 363-377.

Katon, W. J. (2003). Clinical and health services relationships between major depression, depressive symptoms, and general medical illness. *Biological Psychiatry, 54,* 216-226.

Kight, M., Gatchel, R. J., & Wesley, L. (1999). Temporomandibular disorders: Evidence for significant overlap with psychopathology. *Health Psychology, 18,* 177-182.

Korszun, A., Hinderstein, B., & Wong, M. (1996). Comorbidity of depression with chronic facial pain and temporomandibular disorders. *Oral Surgery, Oral Medicine, Oral Pathology, Oral Radiology, & Endodontics, 82,* 496-500.

Kudoh, A., Katagai, H., & Takazawa, T. (2002). Increased postoperative pain scores in chronic depression patients who take antidepressants. *Journal of Clinical Anesthesia, 14,* 421-425.

Lautenbacher, S., & Krieg, J. G. (1994). Pain perception in psychiatric disorders: A review of the literature. *Journal of Psychiatric Research, 28,* 109-122.

Pinerua-Shuhaibar, L., Prieto-Rincon, D., Ferrer, A., Bonilla, E., Maixner, W., & Suarez-Roca, H. (1999). Reduced tolerance and cardiovascular response to ischemic pain in minor depression. *Journal of Affective Disorders, 56,* 119-126.

Polatin, P. B., Kinney, R. K., Gatchel, R. J., Lillo, E., & Mayer, T. G. (1993). Psychiatric illness and chronic low back pain: The mind and the spine—which goes first? *Spine, 18(1),* 66-71.

Radloff, L. (1977). The CES-D scale: A self-report depression scale for research in the general population. *Journal of Applied Psychological Measurement, 1,* 385-401.

Reid, M. C., Guo, Z., Towle, V. R., Kerns, R. D., & Concato, J. (2002). Pain-related disability among older male veterans receiving primary care. *Journal of Gerontology Series A: Biological Sciences and Medical Sciences, 57,* M727-M732.

Robinson, M. E., & Riley, J. L. I. (1999). The role of emotion in pain. In R. J. Gatchel & D. C. Turk (Eds.), *Psychosocial factors in pain* (pp. 74-88). New York: Guilford Press.

Ward, N. G., Bloom, V. L., Dworkin, S., Fawcett, J., Narasimhachari, N., & Friedel, R. O. (1982). Psychobiological markers in coexisting pain and depression: Toward a unified theory. *Journal of Clinical Psychiatry, 43,* 32-41.

Willoughby, S. G., Hailey, B. J., Mulkana, S., & Rowe, J. (2002). The effect of laboratory-induced depressed mood state on responses to pain. *Behavioral Medicine, 28,* 23-31.

Zung, W. W. (1965). A self-rating depression scale. *Archives of General Psychiatry, 12,* 63-70.

Diathesis-stress model

Banks, S. M., & Kerns, R. D. (1996). Explaining high rates of depression in chronic pain: A diathesis-stress framework. *Psychological Bulletin, 119,* 95-110.

Dworkin, R. H. & Banks, S. M. (1999). A vulnerability-diathesis-stress model of chronic pain: Herpes zoster and the development of postherpetic neuralgia. In R. J. Gatchel & D. C. Turk (Eds.), *Psychosocial factors in pain* (pp. 247-269). New York: Guilford Press.

Disability

Arnstein, P. (2000). The mediation of disability by self efficacy in different samples of chronic pain patients. *Disability and Rehabilitation, 22,* 794-801.

Arnstein, P., Caudill, M., Mandle, C. L., Norris, A., & Beasley, R. (1999). Self-efficacy as a mediator of the relationship between pain intensity, disability and depression in chronic pain patients. *Pain, 80,* 483-491.

Barry, L. C., Guo, Z., Kerns, R. D., Duong, B. D., & Reid, M. C. (2003). Functional self-efficacy and pain-related disability among older veterans with chronic pain in a primary care setting. *Pain, 104,* 131-137.

Ciccone, D. S., & Just, N. (2001). Pain expectancy and work disability in patients with acute and chronic pain: A test of the fear avoidance hypothesis. *Journal of Pain, 2,* 181-194.

Evers, A. W., Kraaimaat, F. W., Geenen, R., Jacobs, J. W., & Bijlsma, J. W. (2003). Pain coping and social support as predictors of long-term functional disability and pain in early rheumatoid arthritis. *Behaviour Research and Therapy, 41,* 1295-1310.

Fairbank, J. C., Couper, J., Davies, J. B., & O'Brien, J. P. (1980). The Oswestry low back pain disability questionnaire. *Physiotherapy, 66,* 271-273.

Fairbank, J. C., & Pynsent, P. B. (2000). The Oswestry disability index. *Spine, 25,* 2940-2953.

French, D. J., Holroyd, K. A., Pinell, C., Malinoski, P. T., O'Donnell, F., & Hill, K. R. (2000). Perceived self-efficacy and headache-related disability. *Headache, 40,* 647-656.

Lee, C. E., Simmonds, M. J., Novy, D. M., & Jones, S. (2001). Self-reports and clinician-measured physical function among patients with low back pain: A comparison. *Archives of Physical Medicine and Rehabilitation, 82,* 227-231.

Mannion, A. F., Junge, A., Taimela, S., Muntener, M., Lorenzo, K., & Dvorak, J. (2001). Active therapy for chronic low back pain: Part 3. Factors influencing self-rated disability and its change following therapy. *Spine, 26,* 920-929.

Reid, M. C., Guo, Z., Towle, V. R., Kerns, R. D., & Concato, J. (2002). Pain-related disability among older male veterans receiving primary care. *Journal of Gerontology Series A: Biological Sciences and Medical Sciences, 57,* M727-M732.

Rejeski, W. J., Miller, M. E., Foy, C., Messier, S., & Rapp, S. (2001). Self-efficacy and the progression of functional limitations and self-reported disability in older adults with knee pain. *Journal of Gerontology Series B: Psychological Sciences and Social Sciences, 56,* S261-S265.

Robinson, J. P. (2001). Disability evaluation in painful conditions. In D. C. Turk & R. Melzack (Eds.), *Handbook of pain assessment* (pp. 248-272). New York: Guilford Press.

Roland, M., & Morris, R. (1983a). A study of the natural history of back pain. Part I: Development of a reliable and sensitive measure of disability in low back pain. *Spine, 8,* 141-144.

Roland, M., & Morris, R. (1983b). A study of the natural history of low back pain. Part II: Development of guidelines for trials of treatment in primary care. *Spine, 8,* 145-150.

Simmonds, M. J., Olson, S. L., Jones, S., Hussein, T., Lee, C. E., Novy, D., & Radwan, H. (1998). Psychometric characteristics and clinical usefulness of physical performance tests in patients with low back pain. *Spine, 23,* 2412-2421.

Walsh, D. A., & Radcliffe, J. C. (2002). Pain beliefs and perceived physical disability of patients with chronic low back pain. *Pain, 97,* 23-31.

Distraction

Bantick, S. J., Wise, R. G., Ploghaus, A., Clare, S., Smith, S. M., & Tracey, I. (2002). Imaging how attention modulates pain in humans using functional MRI. *Brain, 125,* 310-319.

Bushnell, M. C. & Duncan, G. H. (1989). Sensory and affective aspects of pain perception: Is medial thalamus restricted to emotional issues? *Experimental Brain Research, 78,* 415-418.

Bushnell, M. C., Duncan, G. H., Dubner, R., & He, L. F. (1984). Activity of trigeminothalamic neurons in medullary dorsal horn of awake monkeys trained in a thermal discrimination task. *Journal of Neurophysiology, 52,* 170-187.

Hoffman, H. G., Patterson, D. R., & Carrougher, G. J. (2000). Use of virtual reality for adjunctive treatment of adult burn pain during physical therapy: A controlled study. *Clinical Journal of Pain, 16,* 244-250.

Hoffman, H. G., Patterson, D. R., Carrougher, G. J., & Sharar, S. R. (2001). Effectiveness of virtual reality-based pain control with multiple treatments. *Clinical Journal of Pain, 17,* 229-235.

Johnson, M. H., Breakwell, G., Douglas, W., & Humphries, S. (1998). The effects of imagery and sensory detection distractors on different measures of pain: How does distraction work? *British Journal of Clinical Psychology, 37,* 141-154.

Lembo, T., Fitzgerald, L., Matin, K., Woo, K., Mayer, E. A., & Naliboff, B. D. (1998). Audio and visual stimulation reduces patient discomfort during screening flexible sigmoidoscopy. *American Journal of Gastroenterology, 93,* 1113-1116.

Longe, S. E., Wise, R., Bantick, S., Lloyd, D., Johansen-Berg, H., McGlone, F., & Tracey, I. (2001). Counter-stimulatory effects on pain perception and processing are significantly altered by attention: An fMRI study. *Neuroreport, 12,* 2021-2025.

McCaul, K. D., & Malott, J. M. (1984). Distraction and coping with pain. *Psychological Bulletin, 95,* 516-533.

McCaul, K. D., Monson, N., & Maki, R. H. (1992). Does distraction reduce pain-produced distress among college students? *Journal of Health Psychology, 11,* 210-217.

Tracey, I., Ploghaus, A., Gati, J. S., Clare, S., Smith, S., Menon, R. S., & Matthews, P. M. (2002). Imaging attentional modulation of pain in the periaqueductal gray in humans. *Journal of Neuroscience, 22,* 2748-2752.

Villemure, C., & Bushnell, M. C. (2002). Cognitive modulation of pain: How do attention and emotion influence pain processing? *Pain, 95,* 195-199.

Dysmenorrhea

Amodei, N., Nelson, R. O., Jarrett, R. B., & Sigmon, S. (1987). Psychological treatments of dysmenorrhea: Differential effectiveness for spasmodics and congestives. *Journal of Behavior Therapy and Experimental Psychiatry, 18,* 95-103.

Bajaj, P., Bajaj, P., Madsen, H., & Arendt-Nielsen, L. (2002). A comparison of modality-specific somatosensory changes during menstruation in dysmenorrheic and nondysmenorrheic women. *Clinical Journal of Pain, 18,* 180-190.

Bancroft, J., Williamson, L., Warner, P., Rennie, D., & Smith, S. K. (1993). Perimenstrual complaints in women complaining of PMS, menorrhagia, and dysmenorrhea: Toward a dismantling of the premenstrual syndrome. *Psychosomatic Medicine, 55,* 133-145.

Banikarim, C., Chacko, M. R., & Kelder, S. H. (2000). Prevalence and impact of dysmenorrhea on Hispanic female adolescents. *Archives of Pediatrics & Adolescent Medicine, 154,* 1226-1229.

Dalton, K. (1969). *The menstrual cycle.* New York: Pantheon Books.

Fillingim, R. B. (2004). Disturbances of pain perception in menstrual cycle-related disorders. In S. Lautenbacher & R. B. Fillingim (Eds.), *Pathophysiology of pain perception* (pp. 133-140). New York: Kluwer Academic.

Freeman, E. W., Rickels, K., & Sondheimer, S. J. (1993). Premenstrual symptoms and dysmenorrhea in relation to emotional distress factors in adolescents. *Journal of Psychosomatic Obstetrics & Gynecology, 14,* 41-50.

Giamberardino, M. A., Berkley, K. J., Iezzi, S., Debigontina, P., & Vecchiet, L. (1997). Pain threshold variations in somatic wall tissues as a function of menstrual cycle, segmental site and tissue depth in non-dysmenorrheic women, dysmenorrheic women and men. *Pain, 71,* 187-197.

Granot, M., Yarnitsky, D., Itskovitz-Eldor, J., Granovsky, Y., Peer, E., & Zimmer, E. Z. (2001). Pain perception in women with dysmenorrhea. *Obstetrics & Gynecology, 98,* 407-411.

Harlow, S. D., & Park, M. (1996). A longitudinal study of risk factors for the occurrence, duration and severity of menstrual cramps in a cohort of college women. *British Journal of Obstetrics and Gynecology, 103,* 1134-1142.

Hillen, T. I., Grbavac, S. L., Johnston, P. J., Straton, J. A., & Keogh, J. M. (1999). Primary dysmenorrhea in young Western Australian women: Prevalence, impact, and knowledge of treatment. *Journal of Adolescent Health, 25,* 40-45.

Zondervan, K. T., Yudkin, P. L., Vessey, M. P., Dawes, M. G., Barlow, D. H., & Kennedy, S. H. (1998). The prevalence of chronic pelvic pain in women in the United Kingdom: A systematic review. *British Journal of Obstetrics and Gynecology, 105,* 93-99.

Education

Allard, P., Maunsell, E., Labbe, J., & Dorval, M. (2001). Educational interventions to improve cancer pain control: A systematic review. *Journal of Palliative Medicine, 4,* 191-203.

Burton, A. K., Waddell, G., Tillotson, K. M., & Summerton, N. (1999). Information and advice to patients with back pain can have a positive effect. A randomized controlled trial of a novel educational booklet in primary care. *Spine, 24,* 2484-2491.

Butler, G. S., Hurley, C. A., Buchanan, K. L., & Smith-VanHorne, J. (1996). Prehospital education: Effectiveness with total hip replacement surgery patients. *Patient Education & Counseling, 29,* 189-197.

Daltroy, L. H., Morlino, C. I., Eaton, H. M., Poss, R., & Liang, M. H. (1998). Preoperative education for total hip and knee replacement patients. *Arthritis Care and Research, 11,* 469-478.

de Wit, R., van Dam, F., Loonstra, S., Zandbelt, L., van Buuren, A., van der, H. K., Leenhouts, G., Duivenvoorden, H., & Huijer Abu-Saad, H. (2001). Improving the quality of pain treatment by a tailored pain education programme for cancer patients in chronic pain. *European Journal of Pain, 5,* 241-256.

Derebery, V. J., Giang, G. M., Saracino, G., & Fógarty, W. T. (2002). Evaluation of the impact of a low back pain educational intervention on physicians' practice patterns and patients' outcomes. *Journal of Occupational and Environmental Medicine, 44,* 977-984.

Ersek, M., Turner, J. A., McCurry, S. M., Gibbons, L., & Kraybill, B. M. (2003). Efficacy of a self-management group intervention for elderly persons with chronic pain. *Clinical Journal of Pain, 19,* 156-167.

Frost, H., Klaber Moffett, J. A., Moser, J. S., & Fairbank, J. C. (1995). Randomised controlled trial for evaluation of fitness programme for patients with chronic low back pain. *British Medical Journal, 310,* 151-154.

Ger, L. P., Lee, M. C., Wong, C. S., Chao, S. S., Wang, J. J., & Ho, S. T. (2003). The effect of education and clinical practice on knowledge enlightenment to and attitudes toward the use of analgesics for cancer pain among physicians and medical students. *Acta Anaesthesiologica Sinica, 41,* 105-114.

Giraudet-Le Quintrec, J. S., Coste, J., Vastel, L., Pacault, V., Jeanne, L., Lamas, J. P., Kerboull, L., Fougeray, M., Conseiller, C., Kahan, A., & Courpied, J. P. (2003). Positive effect of patient education for hip surgery: A randomized trial. *Clinical Orthopaedics & Related Research, September (414),* 112-120.

Haugli, L., Steen, E., Laerum, E., Nygard, R., & Finset, A. (2001). Learning to have less pain—Is it possible? A one-year follow-up study of the effects of a personal construct group learning programme on patients with chronic musculoskeletal pain. *Patient Education & Counseling, 45,* 111-118.

Hazard, R. G., Reid, S., Haugh, L. D., & McFarlane, G. (2000). A controlled trial of an educational pamphlet to prevent disability after occupational low back injury. *Spine, 25,* 1419-1423.

Keefe, F. J., Caldwell, D. S., Baucom, D., Salley, A., Robinson, E., Timmons, K., Beaupre, P., Weisberg, J., & Helms, M. (1996). Spouse-assisted coping skills training in the management of osteoarthritic knee pain. *Arthritis Care & Research, 9,* 279-291.

Keefe, F. J., Caldwell, D. S., Baucom, D., Salley, A., Robinson, E., Timmons, K., Beaupre, P., Weisberg, J., & Helms, M. (1999). Spouse-assisted coping skills training in the management of knee pain in osteoarthritis: Long-term follow-up results. *Arthritis Care & Research, 12,* 101-111.

Koes, B. W., van Tulder, M. W., van der Windt, W. M., & Bouter, L. M. (1994). The efficacy of back schools: A review of randomized clinical trials. *Journal of Clinical Epidemiology, 47,* 851-862.

Linton, S. J., & Andersson, T. (2000). Can chronic disability be prevented? A randomized trial of a cognitive-behavior intervention and two forms of information for patients with spinal pain. *Spine, 25,* 2825-2831.

Maier-Riehle, B., & Harter, M. (2001). The effects of back schools—A meta-analysis. *International Journal of Rehabilitation Research, 24,* 199-206.

Oliver, J. W., Kravitz, R. L., Kaplan, S. H., & Meyers, F. J. (2001). Individualized patient education and coaching to improve pain control among cancer outpatients. *Journal of Clinical Oncology, 19,* 2206-2212.

Ray, W. A., Stein, C. M., Byrd, V., Shorr, R., Pichert, J. W., Gideon, P., Arnold, K., Brandt, K. D., Pincus, T., & Griffin, M. R. (2001). Educational program for physicians to reduce use of non-steroidal anti-inflammatory drugs among community-dwelling elderly persons: A randomized controlled trial. *Medical Care, 39,* 425-435.

Shuldham, C. (1999). A review of the impact of pre-operative education on recovery from surgery. *International Journal of Nursing Studies, 36,* 171-177.

Stein, C. M., Griffin, M. R., Taylor, J. A., Pichert, J. W., Brandt, K. D., & Ray, W. A. (2001). Educational program for nursing home physicians and staff to reduce use of non-steroidal anti-inflammatory drugs among nursing home residents: A randomized controlled trial. *Medical Care, 39,* 436-445.

Ury, W. A., Rahn, M., Tolentino, V., Pignotti, M. G., Yoon, J., McKegney, P., & Sulmasy, D. P. (2002). Can a pain management and palliative care curriculum improve the opioid prescribing practices of medical residents? *Journal of General Internal Medicine, 17,* 625-631.

West, C. M., Dodd, M. J., Paul, S. M., Schumacher, K., Tripathy, D., Koo, P., & Miaskowski, C. (2003). The PRO-SELF(c): Pain Control Program—An effective approach for cancer pain management. *Oncology Nursing Forum, 30,* 65-73.

Emotion

Blumer, D., & Heilbronn, M. (1982). Chronic pain as a variant of depressive disease: The pain-prone disorder. *Journal of Nervous and Mental Disease, 170,* 381-406.

Flor, H., & Turk, D. C. (1989). Psychophysiology of chronic pain: Do chronic pain patients exhibit symptom-specific psychophysiological responses? *Psychology Bulletin, 105,* 215-259.

Robinson, M. E., & Riley, J. L. I. (1999). The role of emotion in pain. In R. J. Gatchel & D. C. Turk (Eds.), *Psychosocial factors in pain* (pp. 74-88). New York: Guilford Press.

Tsigos, C., & Chrousos, G. P. (2002). Hypothalamic-pituitary-adrenal axis, neuroendocrine factors and stress. *Journal of Psychosomatic Research, 53,* 865-871.

Ward, N. G., Bloom, V. L., Dworkin, S., Fawcett, J., Narasimhachari, N., & Friedel, R. O. (1982). Psychobiological markers in coexisting pain and depression: Toward a unified theory. *Journal of Clinical Psychiatry, 43,* 32-41.

Endogenous opioids

Bandura, A., O'Leary, A., Taylor, C. B., Gauthier, J., & Gossard, D. (1987). Perceived self-efficacy and pain control: Opioid and nonopioid mechanisms. *Journal of Personality and Social Psychology, 53,* 563-571.

Basbaum, A. I., & Fields, H. L. (1984). Endogenous pain control systems: Brainstem spinal pathways and endorphin circuitry. *Annual Review of Neuroscience, 7,* 309-338.

Bruehl, S., Burns, J. W., Chung, O. Y., Ward, P., & Johnson, B. (2002). Anger and pain sensitivity in chronic low back pain patients and pain-free controls: The role of endogenous opioids. *Pain, 99,* 223-233.

Frid, M., Singer, G., & Rana, C. (1979). Interactions between personal expectations and naloxone: Effects on tolerance to ischemic pain. *Psychopharmacology, 65,* 225-231.

Hughes, J., Smith, T. W., Kosterlitz, H. W., Fothergill, L. A., & Morgan, B. A. (1975). Identification of two related pentapeptides from the brain with potent opiate agonist activity. *Nature, 258,* 577-579.

Terenius, L. (1975). Effect of peptides and aminoacids on dihydromorphine binding to opiate receptor. *Journal of Pharmacy and Pharmacology, 27,* 450-453.

Ethnicity

Ang, D. C., Ibrahim, S. A., Burant, C. J., Siminoff, L. A., & Kent, K. C. (2002). Ethnic differences in the perception of prayer and consideration of joint arthroplasty. *Medical Care, 40,* 471-476.

Bates, M. S., Edwards, W. T., & Anderson, K. O. (1993). Ethnocultural influences on variation in chronic pain perception. *Pain, 52,* 101-112.

Bhopal, R. (1997). Is research into ethnicity and health racist, unsound, or important science? *British Medical Journal, 314,* 1751-1756.

Bhopal, R. (1998). Spectre of racism in health and health care: Lessons from history and the United States. *British Medical Journal, 316,* 1970-1973.

Bhopal, R., & Rankin, J. (1999). Concepts and terminology in ethnicity, race and health: Be aware of the ongoing debate. *British Dental Journal, 186,* 483-484.

Byrd, W. M., & Clayton, L. A. (2002). Racial and ethnic disparities in healthcare: A background and history. In B. D. Smedley, A. Y. Stith, & A. R. Nelson (Eds.), *Unequal treatment* (pp. 455-527). Washington, DC: The National Academies Press.

Campbell, C. M., Edwards, R. R., & Fillingim, R. B. (2005). Ethnic differences in responses to multiple experimental pain stimuli. *Pain, 113,* 20-26.

Edwards, C. L., Fillingim, R. B., & Keefe, F. J. (2001). Race, ethnicity and pain: A review. *Pain, 94,* 133-137.

Green, C. R., Anderson, K. O., Baker, T. A., Campbell, L. C., Decker, S., Fillingim, R. B., Kaloukalani, D. A., Lasch, K. E., Myers, C., Tait, R. C., Todd, K. H., & Vallerand, A. H. (2003). The unequal burden of pain: Confronting racial and ethnic disparities in pain. *Pain Medicine, 4,* 277-294.

Ibrahim, S. A., Siminoff, L. A., Burant, C. J., & Kwoh, C. K. (2002). Differences in expectations of outcome mediate African American/white patient differences in "willingness" to consider joint replacement. *Arthritis and Rheumatism, 46,* 2429-2435.

Jordan, M. S., Lumley, M. A., & Leisen, J. C. (1998). The relationships of cognitive coping and pain control beliefs to pain and adjustment among African-American and Caucasian women with rheumatoid arthritis. *Arthritis Care & Research, 11,* 80-88.

Rollman, G. B. (1998). Culture and pain. In S. S. Kazarian & D. R. Evans (Eds.), *Cultural clinical psychology: Theory, research, and practice* (pp. 267-286). New York: Oxford University Press.

Zatzick, D. F., & Dimsdale, J. E. (1990). Cultural variations in response to painful stimuli. *Psychosomatic Medicine, 52,* 544-557.

Exercise

Bendix, A. F., Bendix, T., Ostenfeld, S., Bush, E., & Andersen (1995). Active treatment programs for patients with chronic low back pain: A prospective, randomized, observer-blinded study. *European Spine Journal, 4,* 148-152.

Busch, A., Schachter, C. L., Peloso, P. M., & Bombardier, C. (2002). Exercise for treating fibromyalgia syndrome. *The Cochrane Database of Systematic Reviews,* CD003786.

Davis, V. P., Fillingim, R. B., Doleys, D. M., & Davis, M. P. (1992). Assessment of aerobic power in chronic pain patients before and after a multi-disciplinary treatment program. *Archives of Physical Medicine and Rehabilitation, 73,* 726-729.

Droste, C., Greenlee, M. W., Schreck, M., & Roskamm, H. (1991). Experimental pain thresholds and plasma beta-endorphin levels during exercise. *Medicine and Science in Sports and Exercise, 23,* 334-342.

Ettinger, W. H., Jr., Burns, R., Messier, S. P., Applegate, W., Rejeski, W. J., Morgan, T., Shumaker, S., Berry, M. J., O'Toole, M., Monu, J., & Craven, T. (1997). A randomized trial comparing aerobic exercise and resistance exercise with a health education program in older adults with knee osteoarthritis. The Fitness Arthritis and Seniors Trial (FAST). *Journal of the American Medical Association, 277,* 25-31.

Gowans, S. E., de Hueck, A., Voss, S., Silaj, A., Abbey, S. E., & Reynolds, W. J. (2001). Effect of a randomized, controlled trial of exercise on mood and physical function in individuals with fibromyalgia. *Arthritis and Rheumatism, 45,* 519-529.

Gurevich, M., Kohn, P. M., & Davis, C. (1994). Exercise-induced analgesia and the role of reactivity in pain sensitivity. *Journal of Sports Science, 12,* 549-559.

Kemppainen, P., Paalasmaa, P., Pertovaara, A., Alila, A., & Johansson, G. (1990). Dexamethasone attenuates exercise-induced dental analgesia in man. *Brain Research, 519,* 329-332.

Lahad, A., Malter, A. D., Berg, A. O., & Deyo, R. A. (1994). The effectiveness of four interventions for the prevention of low back pain. *Journal of the American Medical Association, 272,* 1286-1291.

Mior, S. (2001). Exercise in the treatment of chronic pain. *Clinical Journal of Pain, 17,* S77-S85.

Nicholas, M. K., Wilson, P. H., & Goyen, J. (1992). Comparison of cognitive-behavioral group treatment and an alternative non-psychological treatment for chronic low back pain. *Pain, 48,* 339-347.

O'Grady, M., Fletcher, J., & Ortiz, S. (2000). Therapeutic and physical fitness exercise prescription for older adults with joint disease: An evidence-based approach. *Rheumatic Diseases Clinics of North America, 26,* 617-646.

Pertovaara, A., Huopaniemi, T., Virtanen, A., & Johansson, G. (1984). The influence of exercise on dental pain thresholds and the release of stress hormones. *Physiology & Behavior, 33,* 923-926.

Richards, S. C. & Scott, D. L. (2002). Prescribed exercise in people with fibromyalgia: Parallel group randomised controlled trial. *British Medical Journal, 325,* 185.

Sculco, A. D., Paup, D. C., Fernhall, B., & Sculco, M. J. (2001). Effects of aerobic exercise on low back pain patients in treatment. *The Spine Journal, 1,* 95-101.

Seraganian, P. (1993). *Exercise psychology: The influence of physical exercise on psychological processes.* New York: John Wiley & Sons.

Sim, J., & Adams, N. (2002). Systematic review of randomized controlled trials of nonpharmacological interventions for fibromyalgia. *Clinical Journal of Pain, 18,* 324-336.

van Tulder, M., Malmivaara, A., Esmail, R., & Koes, B. (2000). Exercise therapy for low back pain: A systematic review within the framework of the cochrane collaboration back review group. *Spine, 25,* 2784-2796.

Williams, D. A. (2003). Psychological and behavioural therapies in fibromyalgia and related syndromes. *Best Practice & Research: Clinical Rheumatology, 17,* 649-665.

Expectancies

Bachiocco, V., Morselli, A. M., & Carli, G. (1993). Self-control expectancy and postsurgical pain: Relationships to previous pain, behavior in past pain, familial pain tolerance models, and personality. *Journal of Pain & Symptom Management, 8,* 205-214.

de Groot, K. I., Boeke, S., & Passchier, J. (1999). Preoperative expectations of pain and recovery in relation to postoperative disappointment in patients undergoing lumbar surgery. *Medical Care, 37,* 149-156.

Lowery, D., Fillingim, R. B., & Wright, R. A. (2003). Sex differences and incentive effects on perceptual and cardiovascular responses to cold pressor pain. *Psychosomatic Medicine, 65,* 284-291.

Mahomed, N. N., Liang, M. H., Cook, E. F., Daltroy, L. H., Fortin, P. R., Fossel, A. H., & Katz, J. N. (2002). The importance of patient expectations in predicting functional outcomes after total joint arthroplasty. *Journal of Rheumatology, 29,* 1273-1279.

Sullivan, M. J., Rodgers, W. M., & Kirsch, I. (2001). Catastrophizing, depression and expectancies for pain and emotional distress. *Pain, 91,* 147-154.

Svensson, I., Sjostrom, B., & Haljamae, H. (2001). Influence of expectations and actual pain experiences on satisfaction with postoperative pain management. *European Journal of Pain, 5,* 125-135.

Thomas, T., Robinson, C., Champion, D., McKell, M., & Pell, M. (1998). Prediction and assessment of the severity of post-operative pain and of satisfaction with management. *Pain, 75,* 177-185.

Wallace, L. M. (1985). Surgical patients' expectations of pain and discomfort: Does accuracy of expectations minimise post-surgical pain and distress? *Pain, 22,* 363-373.

Eye movement desensitization and reprocessing

Grant, M. (2000). EMDR: A new treatment for trauma and chronic pain. *Complementary Therapies in Nursing and Midwifery, 6,* 91-94.

Grant, M., & Threlfo, C. (2002). EMDR in the treatment of chronic pain. *Journal of Clinical Psychology, 58,* 1505-1520.

Herbert, J. D., Lilienfeld, S. O., Lohr, J. M., Montgomery, R. W., O'Donohue, W. T., Rosen, G. M., & Tolin, D. F. (2000). Science and pseudoscience in the development of eye movement desensitization and reprocessing: Implications for clinical psychology. *Clinical Psychology Review, 20,* 945-971.

Lohr, J. M., Lilienfeld, S. O., Tolin, D. F., & Herbert, J. D. (1999). Eye movement desensitization and reprocessing: An analysis of specific versus nonspecific treatment factors. *Journal of Anxiety Disorders, 13,* 185-207.

Shapiro, F., & Maxfield, L. (2002). Eye movement desensitization and reprocessing (EMDR): Information processing in the treatment of trauma. *Journal of Clinical Psychology, 58,* 933-946.

Factitious disorder

American Psychiatric Association (1994). *Diagnostic and statistical manual of mental disorders: DSM-IV* (4th ed.). Washington, DC: American Psychiatric Association.

Family

Barlow, J. H., Cullen, L. A., Foster, N. E., Harrison, K., & Wade, M. (1999). Does arthritis influence perceived ability to fulfill a parenting role? Perceptions of mothers, fathers and grandparents. *Patient Education & Counseling, 37,* 141-151.

Block, A. R., Kremer, E. F., & Gaylor, M. (1980). Behavioral treatment of chronic pain: The spouse as a discriminative cue for pain behavior. *Pain, 9,* 243-252.

Burns, J. W., Johnson, B. J., Mahoney, N., Devine, J., & Pawl, R. (1996). Anger management style, hostility and spouse responses: Gender differences in predictors of adjustment among chronic pain patients. *Pain, 64,* 445-453.

Buskila, D., & Neumann, L. (1997). Fibromyalgia syndrome (FM) and nonarticular tenderness in relatives of patients with FM. *Journal of Rheumatology, 24,* 941-944.

Buskila, D., Neumann, L., Hazanov, I., & Carmi, R. (1996). Familial aggregation in the fibromyalgia syndrome. *Seminars in Arthritis & Rheumatism, 26,* 605-611.

Edwards, P. W., Zeichner, A., Kuczmierczyk, A. R., & Boczkowski, J. (1985). Familial pain models: The relationship between family history of pain and current pain experience. *Pain, 21,* 379-384.

Ehde, D. M., Holm, J. E., & Metzger, D. L. (1991). The role of family structure, functioning, and pain modeling in headache. *Headache, 31,* 35-40.

Fillingim, R. B., Doleys, D. M., Edwards, R. R., & Lowery, D. (2003). Spousal responses are differentially associated with clinical variables in women and men with chronic pain. *Clinical Journal of Pain, 19,* 217-224.

Fillingim, R. B., Edwards, R. R., & Powell, T. (2000). Sex-dependent effects of reported familial pain history on clinical and experimental pain responses. *Pain, 86,* 87-94.

Flor, H., Breitenstein, C., Birbaumer, N., & Furst, M. (1995). A psychophysiological analysis of spouse solicitousness towards pain behaviors, spouse interaction, and pain perception. *Behavior Therapy, 26,* 255-272.

Flor, H., Kerns, R. D., & Turk, D. C. (1987). The role of spouse reinforcement, perceived pain, and activity levels of chronic pain patients. *Journal of Psychosomatic Research, 31,* 251-259.

Flor, H., Lutzenberger, W., Knost, B., Diesch, E., & Birbaumer, N. (2002). Spouse presence alters brain response to pain. Society for Neuroscience, 754.4.

Gil, K. M., Keefe, F. J., Crisson, J. E., & Van Dalfsen, P. J. (1987). Social support and pain behavior. *Pain, 29*(2), 209-217.

Hunfeld, J. A., Perquin, C. W., Duivenvoorden, H. J., Hazebroek-Kampschreur, A. A., Passchier, J., Suijlekom-Smit, L. W., & van der Wouden, J. C. (2001). Chronic pain and its impact on quality of life in adolescents and their families. *Journal of Pediatric Psychology, 26,* 145-153.

Hunfeld, J. A., Perquin, C. W., Hazebroek-Kampschreur, A. A., Passchier, J., Suijlekom-Smit, L. W., & van der Wouden, J. C. (2002). Physically unexplained chronic pain and its impact on children and their families: The mother's perception. *Psychology and Psychotherapy, 75,* 251-260.

Katon, W., Egan, K., & Miller, D. (1985). Chronic pain: Lifetime psychiatric diagnoses and family history. *American Journal of Psychiatry, 142,* 1156-1160.

Keefe, F. J., Caldwell, D. S., Baucom, D., Salley, A., Robinson, E., Timmons, K., Beaupre, P., Weisberg, J., & Helms, M. (1996). Spouse-assisted coping skills training in the management of osteoarthritic knee pain. *Arthritis Care & Research, 9,* 279-291.

Keefe, F. J., Caldwell, D. S., Baucom, D., Salley, A., Robinson, E., Timmons, K., Beaupre, P., Weisberg, J., & Helms, M. (1999). Spouse-assisted coping skills training in the management of knee pain in osteoarthritis: long-term followup results. *Arthritis Care & Research, 12,* 101-111.

Koutantji, M., Pearce, S. A., & Oakley, D. A. (1998). The relationship between gender and family history of pain with current pain experience and awareness of pain in others. *Pain, 77,* 25-31.

Kraaimaat, F. W., Van Dam-Baggen, R. M., & Bijlsma, J. W. (1995). Association of social support and the spouse's reaction with psychological distress in male and female patients with rheumatoid arthritis. *Journal of Rheumatology, 22,* 644-648.

Lester, N., Lefebvre, J. C., & Keefe, F. J. (1994). Pain in young adults: I. Relationship to gender and family pain history. *Clinical Journal of Pain, 10,* 282-289.

Lousberg, R., Schmidt, A. J., & Groenman, N. H. (1992). The relationship between spouse solicitousness and pain behavior: Searching for more experimental evidence. *Pain, 51,* 75-79.

Merlijn, V. P., Hunfeld, J. A., van der Wouden, J. C., Hazebroek-Kampschreur, A. A., Koes, B. W., & Passchier, J. (2003). Psychosocial factors associated with chronic pain in adolescents. *Pain, 101,* 33-43.

Messinger, H. B., Spierings, E. L., Vincent, A. J., & Lebbink, J. (1991). Headache and family history. *Cephalalgia, 11,* 13-18.

Neumann, L., & Buskila, D. (1997). Quality of life and physical functioning of relatives of fibromyalgia patients. *Seminars in Arthritis & Rheumatism, 26,* 834-839.

Ottman, R., Hong, S., & Lipton, R. B. (1993). Validity of family history data on severe headache and migraine. *Neurology, 43,* 1954-1960.

Palermo, T. M. (2000). Impact of recurrent and chronic pain on child and family daily functioning: A critical review of the literature. *Journal of Developmental & Behavioral Pediatrics, 21,* 58-69.

Pellegrino, M. J., Waylonis, G. W., & Sommer, A. (1989). Familial occurrence of primary fibromyalgia. *Archives of Physical Medicine & Rehabilitation, 70,* 61-63.

Romano, J. M., & Schmaling, K. B. (2001). Assessment of couples and families with chronic pain. In D. C. Turk & R. Melzack (Eds.), *Handbook of pain assessment* (pp. 346-361). New York: Guilford Press.

Romano, J. M., Turner, J. A., & Clancy, S. L. (1989). Sex differences in the relationship of pain patient dysfunction to spouse adjustment. *Pain, 39,* 289-295.

Saarijarvi, S., Rytokoski, U., & Karppi, S. L. (1990). Marital satisfaction and distress in chronic low-back pain patients and their spouses. *Clinical Journal of Pain, 6,* 148-152.

Sternbach, R. A. (1986). Survey of pain in the United States: The Nuprin Pain Report. *Clinical Journal of Pain, 2,* 49-53.

Turkat, I. D., Kuczmierczyk, A. R., & Adams, H. E. (1984). An investigation of the aetiology of chronic headache. The role of headache models. *British Journal of Psychiatry, 145,* 665-666.

Williamson, D., Robinson, M. E., & Melamed, B. (1997). Pain behavior, spouse responsiveness, and marital satisfaction in patients with rheumatoid arthritis. *Behavior Modification, 21,* 97-118.

Fatigue

Fishbain, D. A., Cole, B., Cutler, R. B., Lewis, J., Rosomoff, H. L., & Fosomoff, R. S. (2003). Is pain fatiguing? A structured evidence-based review. *Pain Medicine, 4,* 51-62.

Fear avoidance

Fritz, J. M., & George, S. Z. (2002). Identifying psychosocial variables in patients with acute work-related low back pain: The importance of fear-avoidance beliefs. *Physical Therapy, 82,* 973-983.

Fritz, J. M., George, S. Z., & Delitto, A. (2001). The role of fear-avoidance beliefs in acute low back pain: Relationships with current and future disability and work status. *Pain, 94,* 7-15.

George, S. Z., Fritz, J. M., Bialosky, J. E., & Donald, D. A. (2003). The effect of a fear-avoidance-based physical therapy intervention for patients with acute low back pain: Results of a randomized clinical trial. *Spine, 28,* 2551-2560.

Kori, S. H. (1990). Kinesiophobia: A new view of chronic pain behavior. *Pain Management, January/February,* 35-43.

McCracken, L. M., Zayfert, C., & Gross, R. T. (1992). The Pain Anxiety Symptoms Scale: Development and validation of a scale to measure fear of pain. *Pain, 50,* 67-73.

Vlaeyen, J. W., de Jong, J., Geilen, M., Heuts, P. H., & van Breukelen, G. (2001). Graded exposure in vivo in the treatment of pain-related fear: A replicated single-case experimental design in four patients with chronic low back pain. *Behavior Research and Therapy, 39,* 151-166.

Vlaeyen, J. W., de Jong, J., Geilen, M., Heuts, P. H., & van Breukelen, G. (2002). The treatment of fear of movement/(re)injury in chronic low back pain: Further evidence on the effectiveness of exposure in vivo. *Clinical Journal of Pain, 18,* 251-261.

Vlaeyen, J. W., & Linton, S. J. (2000). Fear-avoidance and its consequences in chronic musculoskeletal pain: A state of the art. *Pain, 85,* 317-332.

Waddell, G., Newton, M., Henderson, I., Somerville, D., & Main, C. J. (1993). A Fear-Avoidance Beliefs Questionnaire (FABQ) and the role of fear-avoidance beliefs in chronic low back pain and disability. *Pain, 52,* 157-168.

Fibromyalgia

Aaron, L. A., Bradley, L. A., Alarcon, G. S., Alexander, R. W., Triana-Alexander, M., Martin, M. Y., & Alberts, K. R. (1996). Psychiatric diagnoses in patients with fibromyalgia are related to health care-seeking behavior rather than to illness. *Arthritis and Rheumatism, 39,* 436-445.

Aaron, L. A., Bradley, L. A., Alarcon, G. S., Triana-Alexander, M., Alexander, R. W., Martin, M. Y., & Alberts, K. R. (1997). Perceived physical and emotional trauma as precipitating events in fibromyalgia. Associations with health care seeking and disability status but not pain severity. *Arthritis and Rheumatism, 40,* 453-460.

Bradley, L. A., Alberts, K. R., Alarcon, G. S., Alexander, R. W., Mountz, M. T., Weigent, D. A., Liv, H. G., Blalock, J. E., Aaron, L. A., Alexander, R. W., et al. (1996). Abnormal brain regional cerebral blood flow (rCBF) and cerebrospinal fluid (CSF) levels of substance P (SP) in patients and nonpatients with fibromyalgia (FM). *Arthritis and Rheumatism, 39,* S212.

Fitzcharles, M. A., Costa, D. D., & Poyhia, R. (2003). A study of standard care in fibromyalgia syndrome: a favorable outcome. *Journal of Rheumatology, 30,* 154-159.

Geisser, M. E., Casey, K. L., Brucksch, C. B., Ribbens, C. M., Appleton, B. B., & Crofford, L. J. (2003). Perception of noxious and innocuous heat stimulation among healthy women and women with fibromyalgia: association with mood, somatic focus, and catastrophizing. *Pain, 102,* 243-250.

Gracely, R. H., Petzke, F., Wolf, J. M., & Clauw, D. J. (2002). Functional magnetic resonance imaging evidence of augmented pain processing in fibromyalgia. *Arthritis and Rheumatism, 46,* 1333-1343.

Granges, G., Zilko, P., & Littlejohn, G. O. (1994). Fibromyalgia syndrome: Assessment of the severity of the condition 2 years after diagnosis. *Journal of Rheumatology, 21,* 523-529.

Gur, A., Karakoc, M., Erdogan, S., Nas, K., Cevik, R., & Sarac, A. J. (2002). Regional cerebral blood flow and cytokines in young females with fibromyalgia. *Clinical and Experimental Rheumatology, 20,* 753-760.

Hurtig, I. M., Raak, R. I., Kendall, S. A., Gerdle, B., & Wahren, L. K. (2001). Quantitative sensory testing in fibromyalgia patients and in healthy subjects: Identification of subgroups. *Clinical Journal of Pain, 17,* 316-322.

Kersh, B. C., Bradley, L. A., Alarcon, G. S., Alberts, K. R., Sotolongo, A., Martin, M. Y., Aaron, L. A., Dewaal, D. F., Domino, M. L., Chaplin, W. F., Palardy, N. R., Cianfrini, L. R., & Triana-Alexander, M. (2001). Psychosocial and health status variables independently predict health care seeking in fibromyalgia. *Arthritis and Rheumatism, 45,* 362-371.

Kosek, E., Ekholm, J., & Hansson, P. (1996). Sensory dysfunction in fibromyalgia patients with implications for pathogenic mechanisms. *Pain, 68,* 375-383.

Kosek, E., & Hansson, P. (1997). Modulatory influence on somatosensory perception from vibration and heterotopic noxious conditioning stimulation (HNCS) in fibromyalgia patients and healthy subjects. *Pain, 70,* 41-51.

Lautenbacher, S., & Rollman, G. B. (1997). Possible deficiencies of pain modulation in fibromyalgia. *Clinical Journal of Pain, 13,* 189-196.

Lautenbacher, S., Rollman, G. B., & McCain, G. A. (1994). Multi-method assessment of experimental and clinical pain in patients with fibromyalgia. *Pain, 59,* 45-53.

McDermid, A. J., Rollman, G. B., & McCain, G. A. (1996). Generalized hypervigilance in fibromyalgia: Evidence of perceptual amplification. *Pain, 66,* 133-144.

Mountz, J. M., Bradley, L. A., Modell, J. G., Alexander, R. W., Triana-Alexander, M., Aaron, L. A., Stewart, K. E., Alarcon, G. S., & Mountz, J. D. (1995). Fibromyalgia in women. Abnormalities of regional cerebral blood flow in the thalamus and the caudate nucleus are associated with low pain threshold levels. *Arthritis and Rheumatism, 38,* 926-938.

Nielson, W. R., Walker, C., & McCain, G. A. (1992). Cognitive behavioral treatment of fibromyalgia syndrome: Preliminary findings. *Journal of Rheumatology, 19,* 98-103.

Rossy, L. A., Buckelew, S. P., Dorr, N., Hagglund, K. J., Thayer, J. F., McIntosh, M. J., Hewett, J. E., & Johnson, J. C. (1999). A meta-analysis of fibromyalgia treatment interventions. *Annals of Behavioral Medicine, 21,* 180-191.

Russell, I. J., Orr, M. D., Littman, B., Vipraio, G. A., Alboukrek, D., Michalek, J. E., Lopez, Y., & MacKillip, F. (1994). Elevated cerebrospinal fluid levels of substance P in patients with the fibromyalgia syndrome. *Arthritis and Rheumatism, 37,* 1593-1601.

Sim, J., & Adams, N. (2002). Systematic review of randomized controlled trials of nonpharmacological interventions for fibromyalgia. *Clinical Journal of Pain, 18,* 324-336.

Staud, R. (2002). Evidence of involvement of central neural mechanisms in generating fibromyalgia pain. *Current Rheumatology Reports, 4,* 299-305.

Staud, R., Robinson, M. E., Vierck, C. J., Jr., Cannon, R. C., Mauderli, A. P., & Price, D. D. (2003). Ratings of experimental pain and pain-related negative affect predict clinical pain in patients with fibromyalgia syndrome. *Pain, 105,* 215-222.

Staud, R., Vierck, C. J., Cannon, R. L., Mauderli, A. P., & Price, D. D. (2001). Abnormal sensitization and temporal summation of second pain (wind-up) in patients with fibromyalgia syndrome. *Pain, 91,* 165-175.

Walker, E. A., Keegan, D., Gardner, G., Sullivan, M., Katon, W. J., & Bernstein, D. (1997). Psychosocial factors in fibromyalgia compared with rheumatoid arthritis: I. Psychiatric diagnoses and functional disability. *Psychosomatic Medicine, 59,* 565-571.

White, K. P., & Nielson, W. R. (1995). Cognitive behavioral treatment of fibromyalgia syndrome: A followup assessment. *Journal of Rheumatology, 22,* 717-721.

White, K. P., Nielson, W. R., Harth, M., Ostbye, T., & Speechley, M. (2002). Chronic widespread musculoskeletal pain with or without fibromyalgia: Psychological distress in a representative community adult sample. *Journal of Rheumatology, 29,* 588-594.

White, K. P., Speechley, M., Harth, M., & Ostbye, T. (1999). The London Fibromyalgia Epidemiology Study: The prevalence of fibromyalgia syndrome in London, Ontario. *Journal of Rheumatology, 26,* 1570-1576.

Williams, D. A. (2003). Psychological and behavioural therapies in fibromyalgia and related syndromes. *Best Practice & Research: Clinical Rheumatology, 17,* 649-665.

Wolfe, F., Ross, K., Anderson, J., Russell, I. J., & Hebert, L. (1995). The prevalence and characteristics of fibromyalgia in the general population. *Arthritis and Rheumatism, 38,* 19-28.

Functional assessment

Al Obaidi, S. M., Nelson, R. M., Al Awadhi, S., & Al Shuwaie, N. (2000). The role of anticipation and fear of pain in the persistence of avoidance behavior in patients with chronic low back pain. *Spine, 25,* 1126-1131.

Fishbain, D. A., Cutler, R., Rosomoff, H. L., & Rosomoff, R. S. (1999). Chronic pain disability exaggeration/malingering and submaximal effort research. *Clinical Journal of Pain, 15,* 244-274.

Lackner, J. M., & Carosella, A. M. (1999). The relative influence of perceived pain control, anxiety, and functional self efficacy on spinal function among patients with chronic low back pain. *Spine, 24,* 2254-2260.

Lee, C. E., Simmonds, M. J., Novy, D. M., & Jones, S. (2001). Self-reports and clinician-measured physical function among patients with low back pain: A comparison. *Archives of Physical Medicine and Rehabilitation, 82,* 227-231.

Polatin, P. B., & Mayer, T. G. (2001). Quantification of function in chronic low back pain. In D. C. Turk & R. Melzack (Eds.), *Handbook of pain assessment* (pp. 191-203). New York: Guilford Press.

Reneman, M. F., Jorritsma, W., Schellekens, J. M., & Goeken, L. N. (2002). Concurrent validity of questionnaire and performance-based disability measurements in patients with chronic nonspecific low back pain. *Journal of Occupational Rehabilitation, 12,* 119-129.

Robinson, M. E., & Dannecker, E. A. (2004). Critical issues in the use of muscle testing for the determination of sincerity of effort. *Clinical Journal of Pain, 20,* 392-398.

Ruan, C. M., Haig, A. J., Geisser, M. E., Yamakawa, K., & Buchholz, R. L. (2001). Functional capacity evaluations in persons with spinal disorders: predicting poor outcomes on the Functional Assessment Screening Test (FAST). *Journal of Occupational Rehabilitation, 11,* 119-132.

Simmonds, M. J., Olson, S. L., Jones, S., Hussein, T., Lee, C. E., Novy, D., & Radwan, H. (1998). Psychometric characteristics and clinical usefulness of physical performance tests in patients with low back pain. *Spine, 23,* 2412-2421.

Gate control theory

Melzack, R., & Wall, P. D. (1965). Pain mechanisms: A new theory. *Science, 150,* 971-979.

Gender

Berkley, K. J. (1997). Sex differences in pain. *Behavioral and Brain Sciences, 20,* 371-380.

Burns, J. W., Johnson, B. J., Devine, J., Mahoney, N., & Pawl, R. (1998). Anger management style and the prediction of treatment outcome among male and female chronic pain patients. *Behaviour Research and Therapy, 36,* 1051-1062.

Craft, R. M. (2003). Sex differences in opioid analgesia: From mouse to man. *Clinical Journal of Pain, 19,* 175-186.

Derbyshire, S. W., Nichols, T., Firestone, L., Townsend, D., & Jones, A. (2002). Gender differences in patterns of cerebral activation during equal experience of painful laser stimulation. *Journal of Pain, 3,* 401-411.

Edwards, R. R., Augustson, E., & Fillingim, R. B. (2000). Sex-specific effects of pain-related anxiety on adjustment to chronic pain. *Clinical Journal of Pain, 16,* 46-53.

Edwards, R. R., Augustson, E., & Fillingim, R. B. (2003). Differential relationships retween anxiety and treatment-associated pain reduction among male and female chronic pain patients. *Clinical Journal of Pain, 19,* 208-216.

Ellermeier, W., & Westphal, W. (1995). Gender differences in pain ratings and pupil reactions to painful pressure stimuli. *Pain, 61,* 435-439.

Fillingim, R. B. (2000). *Sex, gender, and pain.* Seattle: IASP Press.

Fillingim, R. B. (2003). Sex-related influences on pain: A review of mechanisms and clinical implications. *Rehabilitation Psychology, 48,* 165-174.

Fillingim, R. B., & Gear, R. W. (2004). Sex differences in opioid analgesia: Clinical and experimental findings. *European Journal of Pain, 8,* 413-425.

Fillingim, R. B., Keefe, F. J., Light, K. C., Booker, D. K., & Maixner, W. (1996). The influence of gender and psychological factors on pain perception. *Journal of Gender, Culture, and Health, 1,* 21-36.

Fillingim, R. B., & Maixner, W. (1995). Gender differences in the responses to noxious stimuli. *Pain Forum, 4,* 209-221.

Fillingim, R. B., Maixner, W., Kincaid, S., & Silva, S. (1998). Sex differences in temporal summation but not sensory-discriminative processing of thermal pain. *Pain, 75,* 121-127.

France, C. R., & Suchowiecki, S. (1999). A comparison of diffuse noxious inhibitory controls in men and women. *Pain, 81,* 77-84.

Hansen, F. R., Bendix, T., Skov, P., Jensen, C. V., Kristensen, J. H., Krohn, L., & Schioeler, H. (1993). Intensive, dynamic back-muscle exercises, conventional physiotherapy, or placebo-control treatment of low-back pain: A randomized, observer-blind trial. *Spine, 18,* 98-108.

Jensen, I. B., Bergstrom, G., Ljungquist, T., Bodin, L., & Nygren, A. L. (2001). A randomized controlled component analysis of a behavioral medicine rehabilitation program for chronic spinal pain: Are the effects dependent on gender? *Pain, 91,* 65-78.

Kankaanpaa, M., Taimela, S., Airaksinen, O., & Hanninen, O. (1999). The efficacy of active rehabilitation in chronic low back pain. Effect on pain intensity, self-experienced disability, and lumbar fatigability. *Spine, 24,* 1034-1042.

Keogh, E., Hatton, K., & Ellery, D. (2000). Avoidance versus focused attention and the perception of pain: Differential effects for men and women. *Pain, 85,* 225-230.

Krogstad, B. S., Jokstad, A., Dahl, B. L., & Vassend, O. (1996). The reporting of pain, somatic complaints, and anxiety in a group of patients with TMD before and 2 years after treatment: Sex differences. *Journal of Orofacial Pain, 10,* 263-269.

LeResche, L. (1999). Gender considerations in the epidemiology of chronic pain. In I. K. Crombie (Ed.), *Epidemiology of pain* (pp. 43-52). Seattle: IASP Press.

Mannion, A. F., Junge, A., Taimela, S., Muntener, M., Lorenzo, K., & Dvorak, J. (2001). Active therapy for chronic low back pain: Part 3. Factors influencing self-rated disability and its change following therapy. *Spine, 26,* 920-929.

Naliboff, B. D., Berman, S., Chang, L., Derbyshire, S. W., Suyenobu, B., Vogt, B. A., Mandelkern, M., & Mayer, E. A. (2003). Sex-related differences in IBS patients: Central processing of visceral stimuli. *Gastroenterology, 124,* 1738-1747.

Paulson, P. E., Minoshima, S., Morrow, T. J., & Casey, K. L. (1998). Gender differences in pain perception and patterns of cerebral activation during noxious heat stimulation in humans. *Pain, 76,* 223-229.

Riley, J. L., Robinson, M. E., Wise, E. A., Myers, C. D., & Fillingim, R. B. (1998). Sex differences in the perception of noxious experimental stimuli: A meta-analysis. *Pain, 74,* 181-187.

Sarlani, E., & Greenspan, J. D. (2002). Gender differences in temporal summation of mechanically evoked pain. *Pain, 97,* 163-169.

Sternberg, W. F., Bokat, C., Kass, L., Alboyadjian, A., & Gracely, R. H. (2001). Sex-dependent components of the analgesia produced by athletic competition. *Journal of Pain, 2,* 65-74.

Unruh, A. M. (1996). Gender variations in clinical pain experience. *Pain, 65,* 123-167.

Genetics

Aromaa, M., Sillanpaa, M., Rautava, P., & Helenius, H. (2000). Pain experience of children with headache and their families: A controlled study. *Pediatrics, 106,* 270-275.

Bouchard, T. J., Jr., & McGue, M. (2003). Genetic and environmental influences on human psychological differences. *Journal of Neurobiology, 54,* 4-45.

Buskila, D., & Neumann, L. (1997). Fibromyalgia syndrome (FM) and nonarticular tenderness in relatives of patients with FM. *Journal of Rheumatology, 24,* 941-944.

Buskila, D., Neumann, L., Hazanov, I., & Carmi, R. (1996). Familial aggregation in the fibromyalgia syndrome. *Seminars in Arthritis & Rheumatism, 26,* 605-611.

Edwards, P. W., Zeichner, A., Kuczmierczyk, A. R., & Boczkowski, J. (1985). Familial pain models: The relationship between family history of pain and current pain experience. *Pain, 21,* 379-384.

Ehde, D. M., Holm, J. E., & Metzger, D. L. (1991). The role of family structure, functioning, and pain modeling in headache. *Headache, 31,* 35-40.

Eid, M., Riemann, R., Angleitner, A., & Borkenau, P. (2003). Sociability and positive emotionality: Genetic and environmental contributions to the covariation between different facets of extraversion. *Journal of Personality, 71,* 319-346.

Exton, M. S., Artz, M., Siffert, W., & Schedlowski, M. (2003). G protein beta3 subunit 825T allele is associated with depression in young, healthy subjects. *Neuroreport, 14,* 531-533.

Kalantar, J. S., Locke, G. R., III, Talley, N. J., Zinsmeister, A. R., Fett, S. L., & Melton, L. J., III (2003). Is irritable bowel syndrome more likely to be persistent in those with relatives who suffer from gastrointestinal symptoms? A population-based study at three time points. *Alimentary Pharmacology & Therapeutics, 17,* 1389-1397.

Kalantar, J. S., Locke, G. R., III, Zinsmeister, A. R., Beighley, C. M., & Talley, N. J. (2003). Familial aggregation of irritable bowel syndrome: A prospective study. *Gut, 52,* 1703-1707.

Katon, W., Egan, K., & Miller, D. (1985). Chronic pain: Lifetime psychiatric diagnoses and family history. *American Journal of Psychiatry, 142,* 1156-1160.

Kim, H., Neubert, J. K., Iadarola, M. J., San Miguelle, A., Goldman, D., & Dionne, R. A. (2003). Genetic influence on pain sensitivity in humans: Evidence of heritability related to single nucleotide polymorphism (SNP) in opioid receptor genes. In J. O. Dostrovsky, D. B. Carr, & M. Koltzenburg (Eds.), *Proceedings of the 10th World Congress on Pain* (pp. 513-520). Seattle: IASP Press.

Koutantji, M., Pearce, S. A., & Oakley, D. A. (1998). The relationship between gender and family history of pain with current pain experience and awareness of pain in others. *Pain, 77,* 25-31.

Lester, N., Lefebvre, J. C., & Keefe, F. J. (1994). Pain in young adults: I. Relationship to gender and family pain history. *Clinical Journal of Pain, 10,* 282-289.

Levy, R. L., Jones, K. R., Whitehead, W. E., Feld, S. I., Talley, N. J., & Corey, L. A. (2001). Irritable bowel syndrome in twins: Heredity and social learning both contribute to etiology. *Gastroenterology, 121,* 799-804.

Macgregor, A. J., Griffiths, G. O., Baker, J., & Spector, T. D. (1997). Determinants of pressure pain threshold in adult twins: Evidence that shared environmental influences predominate. *Pain, 73,* 253-257.

Messinger, H. B., Spierings, E. L., Vincent, A. J., & Lebbink, J. (1991). Headache and family history. *Cephalalgia, 11,* 13-18.

Mogil, J. S. (1999). The genetic mediation of individual differences in sensitivity to pain and its inhibition. *Proceedings of the National Academy of Sciences USA, 96,* 7744-7751.

Mogil, J. S., Richards, S. P., O'Toole, L. A., Helms, M. L., Mitchell, S. R., & Belknap, J. K. (1997). Genetic sensitivity to hot-plate nociception in DBA/2J and C57BL/6J inbred mouse strains: Possible sex-specific mediation by delta2-opioid receptors. *Pain, 70,* 267-277.

Offenbaecher, M., Bondy, B., de Jonge, S., Glatzeder, K., Kruger, M., Schoeps, P., & Ackenheil, M. (1999). Possible association of fibromyalgia with a polymorphism in the serotonin transporter gene regulatory region. *Arthritis and Rheumatism, 42,* 2482-2488.

Ottman, R., Hong, S., & Lipton, R. B. (1993). Validity of family history data on severe headache and migraine. *Neurology, 43,* 1954-1960.

Pellegrino, M. J., Waylonis, G. W., & Sommer, A. (1989). Familial occurrence of primary fibromyalgia. *Archives of Physical Medicine & Rehabilitation, 70,* 61-63.

Sternbach, R. A. (1986). Survey of pain in the United States: The Nuprin Pain Report. *Clinical Journal of Pain, 2,* 49-53.

Turkat, I. D., Kuczmierczyk, A. R., & Adams, H. E. (1984). An investigation of the aetiology of chronic headache. The role of headache models. *British Journal of Psychiatry, 145,* 665-666.

Zubieta, J. K., Heitzeg, M. M., Smith, Y. R., Bueller, J. A., Xu, K., Xu, Y., Koeppe, R. A., Stohler, C. S., & Goldman, D. (2003). COMT val158met genotype affects mu-opioid neurotransmitter responses to a pain stressor. *Science, 299,* 1240-1243.

Group therapy

Keefe, F. J., Beaupre, P. M., & Gil, K. M. (1996). Group therapy for patients with chronic pain. In R. J. Gatchel and D. C. Turk (Eds.), *Psychological approaches to pain management: A practitioner's handbook* (pp. 259-282). New York: Guilford Press.

Yalom, I. (1985). *The theory and practice of group psychotherapy* (3rd ed.). New York: Basic Books.

Headache

Breslau, N., Lipton, R. B., Stewart, W. F., Schultz, L. R., & Welch, K. M. (2003). Comorbidity of migraine and depression: Investigating potential etiology and prognosis. *Neurology, 60,* 1308-1312.

Breslau, N., Schultz, L. R., Stewart, W. F., Lipton, R. B., Lucia, V. C., & Welch, K. M. (2000). Headache and major depression: Is the association specific to migraine? *Neurology, 54,* 308-313.

Breslau, N., Schultz, L. R., Stewart, W. F., Lipton, R., & Welch, K. M. (2001). Headache types and panic disorder: Directionality and specificity. *Neurology, 56,* 350-354.

Diener, H. C., & Katsarava, Z. (2001). Medication overuse headache. *Current Medical Research & Opinion, 17,* (Supplement 1), s17-s21.

Eccleston, C., Yorke, L., Morley, S., Williams, A. C., & Mastroyannopoulou, K. (2003). Psychological therapies for the management of chronic and recurrent pain in children and adolescents. *The Cochrane Database of Systematic Reviews,* CD003968.

Fernandez, E., & Sheffield, J. (1996). Relative contributions of life events versus daily hassles to the frequency and intensity of headaches. *Headache, 36,* 595-602.

Fritsche, G., & Diener, H. C. (2002). Medication overuse headaches—What is new? *Expert Opinion on Drug Safety, 1,* 331-338.

Haddock, C. K., Rowan, A. B., Andrasik, F., Wilson, P. G., Talcott, G. W., & Stein, R. J. (1997). Home-based behavioral treatments for chronic benign headache: A meta-analysis of controlled trials. *Cephalalgia, 17,* 113-118.

Hasse, L. A., Ritchey, P. N., & Smith, R. (2002). Predicting the number of headache visits by type of patient seen in family practice. *Headache, 42,* 738-746.

Headache Classification Committee of the International Headache Society (1988). Classification and diagnostic criteria for headache disorders, cranial neuralgias and facial pain. *Cephalalgia, 8* (Supplement 7), 1-96.

Headache Classification Committee of the International Headache Society (2004). International classisification of headache disorders, cranial neuralgias and facial pain. *Cephalalgia, 24* (Supplement 1), 1-151.

Ho, K. H., & Ong, B. K. (2003). A community-based study of headache diagnosis and prevalence in Singapore. *Cephalalgia, 23,* 6-13.

Holroyd, K. A., & Lipchik, G. L. (1999). Psychological management of recurrent headache disorders: progress and prospects. In R. J. Gatchel & D. C. Turk (Eds.), *Psychosocial factors in pain* (pp. 193-212). New York: Guilford Press.

Holroyd, K. A., & Penzien, D. B. (1990). Pharmacological versus non-pharmacological prophylaxis of recurrent migraine headache: A meta-analytic review of clinical trials. *Pain, 42,* 1-13.

Jensen, R. (2003). Diagnosis, Epidemiology, and Impact of Tension-type Headache. *Current Pain and Headache Reports, 7,* 455-459.

Limmroth, V., Katsarava, Z., Fritsche, G., Przywara, S., & Diener, H. C. (2002). Features of medication overuse headache following overuse of different acute headache drugs. *Neurology, 59,* 1011-1014.

Lipchik, G. L., Holroyd, K. A., & Nash, J. M. (2002). Cognitive-behavioral management of recurrent headache disorders: A minimal-therapist-contact approach. In D. C. Turk & R. J. Gatchel (Eds.), *Psychological approaches to pain management: A practitioner's handbook* (2nd ed., pp. 365-389). New York: Guilford Press.

Lipton, R. B., Scher, A. I., Kolodner, K., Liberman, J., Steiner, T. J., & Stewart, W. F. (2002). Migraine in the United States: Epidemiology and patterns of health care use. *Neurology, 58,* 885-894.

Lipton, R. B., Stewart, W. F., Diamond, S., Diamond, M. L., & Reed, M. (2001). Prevalence and burden of migraine in the United States: Data from the American Migraine Study II. *Headache, 41,* 646-657.

McCaig, L. F., & Burt, C. W. (2003). National Hospital Ambulatory Medical Care Survey: 2001 emergency department summary. *Advance Data,* 1-29.

Puca, F., Genco, S., Prudenzano, M. P., Savarese, M., Bussone, G., D'Amico, D., Cerbo, R., Gala, C., Coppola, M. T., Gallai, V., Firenze, C., Sarchielli, P., Guazzelli, M., Guidetti, V., Manzoni, G., Granella, F., Muratorio, A., Bonuccelli, U., Nuti, A., Nappi, G., Sandrini, G., Verri, A. P., Sicuteri, F., & Marabini, S. (1999). Psychiatric comorbidity and psychosocial stress in patients with tension-type headache from headache centers in Italy. The Italian Collaborative Group for the Study of Psychopathological Factors in Primary Headaches. *Cephalalgia, 19,* 159-164.

Rasmussen, B. K. (1993). Migraine and tension-type headache in a general population: Precipitating factors, female hormones, sleep pattern and relation to lifestyle. *Pain, 53,* 65-72.

Schwartz, B. S., Stewart, W. F., Simon, D., & Lipton, R. B. (1998). Epidemiology of tension-type headache. *Journal of the American Medical Association, 279,* 381-383.

Silberstein, S. D., Lipton, R. B., & Breslau, N. (1995). Migraine: Association with personality characteristics and psychopathology. *Cephalalgia, 15,* 358-369.

Hyperalgesia

Merskey, H., & Bogduk, N. (1994). *Classification of chronic pain* (2nd ed.). Seattle: IASP Press.

Hypertension

Bruehl, S., Carlson, C. R., & McCubbin, J. A. (1992). The relationship between pain sensitivity and blood pressure in normotensives. *Pain, 48,* 463-467.

Bruehl, S., McCubbin, J. A., & Harden, R. N. (1999). Theoretical review: Altered pain regulatory systems in chronic pain. *Neuroscience & Biobehavioral Reviews, 23,* 877-890.

Fillingim, R. B., Browning, A. D., Powell, T., & Wright, R. A. (2002). Sex differences in perceptual and cardiovascular responses to pain: The influence of a perceived ability manipulation. *Journal of Pain, 3,* 439-445.

Fillingim, R. B., & Maixner, W. (1996). The influence of resting blood pressure and gender on pain repsonses. *Psychosomatic Medicine, 58,* 326-332.

France, C. R. (1999). Decreased pain perception and risk for hypertension: Considering a common physiological mechanism. *Psychophysiology, 36,* 683-692.

Ghione, S. (1996). Hypertension-associated hypalgesia. Evidence in experimental animals and humans, pathophysiological mechanisms, and potential clinical consequences. *Hypertension, 28,* 494-504.

Lowery, D., Fillingim, R. B., & Wright, R. A. (2003). Sex differences and incentive effects on perceptual and cardiovascular responses to cold pressor pain. *Psychosomatic Medicine, 65,* 284-291.

Maixner, W., Fillingim, R., Kincaid, S., Sigurdsson, A., & Harris, M. B. (1997). Relationship between pain sensitivity and resting arterial blood pressure in patients with painful temporomandibular disorders. *Psychosomatic Medicine, 59,* 503-511.

Maixner, W., Touw, K. B., Brody, M. J., Gebhart, G. F., & Long, J. P. (1982). Factors influencing the altered pain perception in the spontaneously hypertensive rat. *Brain Research, 237,* 137-145.

Zamir, N., & Segal, M. (1979). Hypertension-induced analgesia: changes in pain sensitivity in experimental hypertensive rats. *Brain Research, 160,* 170-173.

Zamir, N., Segal, M., & Simantov, R. (1980). Pain sensitivity and opioid activity in genetically and experimentally hypertensive rats. *Brain Research, 184,* 299-310.

Zamir, N., & Shuber, H. (1980). Altered pain perception in hypertensive humans. *Brain Research, 201,* 471-474.

Hypervigilance

Chapman, C. R. (1978). Pain: The perception of noxious events. In R. A. Sternbach (Ed.), *The psychology of pain* (pp. 169-202). New York: Raven Press.

Eccleston, C., Crombez, G., Aldrich, S., & Stannard, C. (1997). Attention and somatic awareness in chronic pain. *Pain, 72,* 209-215.

McBeth, J., Macfarlane, G. J., Benjamin, S., & Silman, A. J. (2001). Features of somatization predict the onset of chronic widespread pain: Results of a large population-based study. *Arthritis and Rheumatism, 44,* 940-946.

McBeth, J., Macfarlane, G. J., Hunt, I. M., & Silman, A. J. (2001). Risk factors for persistent chronic widespread pain: A community-based study. *Rheumatology, 40,* 95-101.

McCracken, L. M. (1997). "Attention" to pain in persons with chronic pain: A behavioural approach. *Behavior Therapy, 28,* 271-284.

McDermid, A. J., Rollman, G. B., & McCain, G. A. (1996). Generalized hypervigilance in fibromyalgia: Evidence of perceptual amplification. *Pain, 66,* 133-144.

Pennebaker, J. W. (1982). *The psychology of physical symptoms.* New York: Springer-Verlag.

Roelofs, J., Peters, M. L., McCracken, L., & Vlaeyen, J. W. (2003). The pain vigilance and awareness questionnaire (PVAQ): Further psychometric evaluation in fibromyalgia and other chronic pain syndromes. *Pain, 101,* 299-306.

Hypnosis

Astin, J. A. (2004). Mind-body therapies for the management of pain. *Clinical Journal of Pain, 20,* 27-32.

Barber, J. (1996). A brief introduction to hypnotic analgesia. In J. Barber (Ed.), *Hypnosis and suggestion in the treatment of pain* (pp. 3-32). New York: W.W. Norton.

Faymonville, M. E., Laureys, S., Degueldre, C., DelFiore, G., Luxen, A., Franck, G., Lamy, M., & Maquet, P. (2000). Neural mechanisms of antinociceptive effects of hypnosis. *Anesthesiology, 92,* 1257-1267.

Faymonville, M. E., Mambourg, P. H., Joris, J., Vrijens, B., Fissette, J., Albert, A., & Lamy, M. (1997). Psychological approaches during conscious sedation. Hypnosis versus stress reducing strategies: A prospective randomized study. *Pain, 73,* 361-367.

Holden, E. W., Deichmann, M. M., & Levy, J. D. (1999). Empirically supported treatments in pediatric psychology: Recurrent pediatric headache. *Journal of Pediatric Psychology, 24,* 91-109.

Kiernan, B. D., Dane, J. R., Phillips, L. H., & Price, D. D. (1995). Hypnotic analgesia reduces R-III nociceptive reflex: further evidence concerning the multifactorial nature of hypnotic analgesia. *Pain, 60,* 39-47.

Montgomery, G. H., DuHamel, K. N., & Redd, W. H. (2000). A meta-analysis of hypnotically induced analgesia: How effective is hypnosis? *International Journal of Clinical & Experimental Hypnosis, 48,* 138-153.

Pan, C. X., Morrison, R. S., Ness, J., Fugh-Berman, A., & Leipzig, R. M. (2000). Complementary and alternative medicine in the management of pain, dyspnea, and nausea and vomiting near the end of life. A systematic review. *Journal of Pain and Symptom Management, 20,* 374-387.

Patterson, D. R., & Jensen, M. P. (2003). Hypnosis and clinical pain. *Psychology Bulletin, 129,* 495-521.

Rainville, P., Duncan, G. H., Price, D. D., Carrier, B., & Bushnell, M. C. (1997). Pain affect encoded in human anterior cingulate but not somatosensory cortex. *Science, 277,* 968-971.

Rainville, P., Hofbauer, R. K., Paus, T., Duncan, G. H., Bushnell, M. C., & Price, D. D. (1999). Cerebral mechanisms of hypnotic induction and suggestion. *Journal of Cognitive Neuroscience, 11,* 110-125.

Sellick, S. M., & Zaza, C. (1998). Critical review of 5 nonpharmacologic strategies for managing cancer pain. *Cancer Prevention and Control, 2,* 7-14.

Hypochondriasis

American Psychiatric Association (1994). *Diagnostic and statistical manual of mental disorders: DSM-IV* (4th ed.). Washington, DC: American Psychiatric Association.

Rief, W., Hessel, A., & Braehler, E. (2001). Somatization symptoms and hypochondriacal features in the general population. *Psychosomatic Medicine, 63,* 595-602.

Irritable bowel syndrome

Blanchard, E. B., & Scharff, L. (2002). Psychosocial aspects of assessment and treatment of irritable bowel syndrome in adults and recurrent abdominal pain in children. *Journal of Consulting and Clinical Psychology, 70,* 725-738.

Bouin, M., Meunier, P., Riberdy-Poitras, M., & Poitras, P. (2001). Pain hypersensitivity in patients with functional gastrointestinal disorders: A gastrointestinal-specific defect or a general systemic condition? *Digestive Diseases & Sciences, 46,* 2542-2548.

Boyce, P. M., Talley, N. J., Balaam, B., Koloski, N. A., & Truman, G. (2003). A randomized controlled trial of cognitive behavior therapy, relaxation training, and routine clinical care for the irritable bowel syndrome. *American Journal of Gastroenterology, 98,* 2209-2218.

Chang, L., Mayer, E. A., Johnson, T., FitzGerald, L. Z., & Naliboff, B. (2000). Differences in somatic perception in female patients with irritable bowel syndrome with and without fibromyalgia. *Pain, 84,* 297-307.

Creed, F., Fernandes, L., Guthrie, E., Palmer, S., Ratcliffe, J., Read, N., Rigby, C., Thompson, D., & Tomenson, B. (2003). The cost-effectiveness of psychotherapy and paroxetine for severe irritable bowel syndrome. *Gastroenterology, 124,* 303-317.

Drossman, D. A. (1999). Do psychosocial factors define symptom severity and patient status in irritable bowel syndrome? *The American Journal of Medicine, 107,* 41S-50S.

Drossman, D. A., Whitehead, W. E., & Camilleri, M. (1997). Irritable bowel syndrome: A technical review for practice guideline development. *Gastroenterology, 112,* 2120-2137.

Gwee, K. A., Graham, J. C., McKendrick, M. W., Collins, S. M., Marshall, J. S., Walters, S. J., & Read, N. W. (1996). Psychometric scores and persistence of irritable bowel after infectious diarrhoea. *Lancet, 347,* 150-153.

Gwee, K. A., Leong, Y. L., Graham, C., McKendrick, M. W., Collins, S. M., Walters, S. J., Underwood, J. E., & Read, N. W. (1999). The role of psychological and biological factors in postinfective gut dysfunction. *Gut, 44,* 400-406.

Koloski, N. A., Talley, N. J., & Boyce, P. M. (2001). Predictors of health care seeking for irritable bowel syndrome and nonulcer dyspepsia: A critical review of the literature on symptom and psychosocial factors. *American Journal of Gastroenterology, 96,* 1340-1349.

Mayer, E. A., Craske, M., & Naliboff, B. D. (2001). Depression, anxiety, and the gastrointestinal system. *Journal of Clinical Psychiatry, 62* (Supplement 8), 28-36.

Mayer, E. A., & Gebhart, G. F. (1994). Basic and clinical aspects of visceral hyperalgesia. *Gastroenterology, 107,* 271-293.

Mertz, H., Naliboff, B., Munakata, J., Niazi, N., & Mayer, E. A. (1995). Altered rectal perception is a biological marker of patients with irritable bowel syndrome. *Gastroenterology, 109,* 40-52.

Naliboff, B. D., Balice, G., & Mayer, E. A. (1998). Psychosocial moderators of quality of life in irritable bowel syndrome. *European Journal of Surgery,* 57-59.

Talley, N. J. (1999). Irritable bowel syndrome: Definition, diagnosis and epidemiology. *Baillieres Best Practice and Research in Clinical Gastroenterology, 13,* 371-384.

Thompson, W. G., Longstreth, G. F., Drossman, D. A., Heaton, K. W., Irvine, E. J., & Muller-Lissner, S. A. (1999). Functional bowel disorders and functional abdominal pain. *Gut, 45* (Supplement 2), II43-II47.

Verne, G. N., Robinson, M. E., & Price, D. D. (2001). Hypersensitivity to visceral and cutaneous pain in the irritable bowel syndrome. *Pain, 93,* 7-14.

Whitehead, W. E., Crowell, M. D., Robinson, J. C., Heller, B. R., & Schuster, M. M. (1992). Effects of stressful life events on bowel symptoms: Subjects with irritable bowel syndrome compared with subjects without bowel dysfunction. *Gut, 33,* 825-830.

Whitehead, W. E., Palsson, O., & Jones, K. R. (2002). Systematic review of the comorbidity of irritable bowel syndrome with other disorders: What are the causes and implications? *Gastroenterology, 122,* 1140-1156.

Language

Clark, W. C., Fletcher, J. D., Janal, M. N., & Carroll, J. D. (1995). Hierarchical clustering of 270 pain/emotion descriptors: Toward a revision of the McGill Pain Questionnaire. In B. Bromm & J. Desmedt (Eds.), *Pain and the brain: From nociception to sensation* (pp. 319-330). New York: Raven Press.

Clark, W. C., Kuhl, J. P., Keohan, M. L., Knotkova, H., Winer, R. T., & Griswold, G. A. (2003). Factor analysis validates the cluster structure of the dendrogram underlying the Multidimensional Affect and Pain Survey (MAPS) and challenges the a priori classification of the descriptors in the McGill Pain Questionnaire (MPQ). *Pain, 106,* 357-363.

Kramer, B. J., Harker, J. O., & Wong, A. L. (2002). Descriptions of joint pain by American Indians: Comparison of inflammatory and noninflammatory arthritis. *Arthritis and Rheumatism, 47,* 149-154.

Mauro, G., Tagliaferro, G., Montini, M., & Zanolla, L. (2001). Diffusion model of pain language and quality of life in orofacial pain patients. *Journal of Orofacial Pain, 15,* 36-46.

Moore, R., Brodsgaard, I., Miller, M. L., Mao, T. K., & Dworkin, S. F. (1997). Consensus analysis: Reliability, validity, and informant accuracy in use of American and Mandarin Chinese pain descriptors. *Annals of Behavioral Medicine, 19,* 295-300.

Tammaro, S., Berggren, U., & Bergenholtz, G. (1997). Representation of verbal pain descriptors on a visual analogue scale by dental patients and dental students. *European Journal of Oral Science, 105,* 207-212.

Legal issues

Cassidy, J. D., Carroll, L., Cote, P., Berglund, A., & Nygren, A. (2003). Low back pain after traffic collisions: A population-based cohort study. *Spine, 28,* 1002-1009.

Cassidy, J. D., Carroll, L. J., Cote, P., Lemstra, M., Berglund, A., & Nygren, A. (2000). Effect of eliminating compensation for pain and suffering on the outcome of insurance claims for whiplash injury. *New England Journal of Medicine, 342,* 1179-1186.

Epker, J., & Block, A. R. (2001). Presurgical psychological screening in back pain patients: A review. *Clinical Journal of Pain, 17,* 200-205.

Main, C. J. (1999). Medicolegal aspects of pain: the nature of psychological opinion in cases of personal injury. In R. J. Gatchel & D. C. Turk (Eds.), *Psychosocial factors in pain* (pp. 132-147). New York: Guilford Press.

Rainville, J., Sobel, J. B., Hartigan, C., & Wright, A. (1997). The effect of compensation involvement on the reporting of pain and disability by patients referred for rehabilitation of chronic low back pain. *Spine, 22,* 2016-2024.

Tollison, C. D., Satterthwaite, J. R., Kriegel, M. L., & Hinnant, D. W. (1990). Inter-disciplinary treatment of low back pain. A clinical outcome comparison of compensated versus noncompensated groups. *Orthopedic Reviews, 19,* 701-706.

Zacny, J., Bigelow, G., Compton, P., Foley, K., Iguchi, M., & Sannerud, C. (2003). College on Problems of Drug Dependence taskforce on prescription opioid non-medical use and abuse: Position statement. *Drug & Alcohol Dependence, 69,* 215-232.

Malingering

American Psychiatric Association (1994). *Diagnostic and statistical manual of mental disorders: DSM-IV* (4th ed.). Washington, DC: American Psychiatric Association.

Butcher, J. N., Arbisi, P. A., Atlis, M. M., & McNulty, J. L. (2003). The construct validity of the Lees-Haley Fake Bad Scale: Does this scale measure somatic ma-lingering and feigned emotional distress? *Archives of Clinical Neuropsychology, 18,* 473-485.

Fishbain, D. A., Cutler, R., Rosomoff, H. L., & Rosomoff, R. S. (1999). Chronic pain disability exaggeration/malingering and submaximal effort research. *Clinical Journal of Pain, 15,* 244-274.

McGuire, B. E., Harvey, A. G., & Shores, E. A. (2001). Simulated malingering in pain patients: A study with the Pain Patient Profile. *British Journal of Clinical Psychology, 40,* 71-79.

McGuire, B. E., & Shores, E. A. (2001). Simulated pain on the symptom checklist 90-Revised. *Journal of Clinical Psychology, 57,* 1589-1596.

Robinson, M. E., & Dannecker, E. A. (2004). Critical issues in the use of muscle testing for the determination of sincerity of effort. *Clinical Journal of Pain, 20,* 392-398.

McGill Pain Questionnaire

Clark, W. C., Kuhl, J. P., Keohan, M. L., Knotkova, H., Winer, R. T., & Griswold, G. A. (2003). Factor analysis validates the cluster structure of the dendrogram underlying the Multidimensional Affect and Pain Survey (MAPS) and challenges the a priori classification of the descriptors in the McGill Pain Questionnaire (MPQ). *Pain, 106,* 357-363.

Fernandez, E., & Boyle, G. J. (2001). Affective and evaluative descriptors of pain in the McGill Pain Questionnaire: Reduction and reorganization. *Journal of Pain, 2,* 318-325.

Melzack, R. (1975). The McGill Pain Questionnaire: Major properties and scoring methods. *Pain, 1,* 277-299.

Melzack, R. (1987). The short-form McGill Pain Questionnaire. *Pain, 30,* 191-197.

Melzack, R. & Katz, J. (2001). The McGill Pain Questionnaire: Appraisal and current status. In D. C. Turk & R. Melzack (Eds.), *Handbook of pain assessment* (pp. 35-52). New York: Guilford Press.

Melzack, R., & Torgerson, W. S. (1971). On the language of pain. *Anesthesiology, 34,* 50-59.

Turk, D. C., Rudy, T. E., & Salovey, P. (1985). The McGill Pain Questionnaire reconsidered: Confirming the factor structure and examining appropriate uses. *Pain, 21,* 385-397.

Memory for pain

Erskine, A., Morley, S., & Pearce, S. (1990). Memory for pain: A review. *Pain, 41,* 255-265.

Everts, B., Karlson, B., Wahrborg, P., Abdon, N., Herlitz, J., & Hedner, T. (1999). Pain recollection after chest pain of cardiac origin. *Cardiology, 92,* 115-120.

Gedney, J. J., Logan, H., & Baron, R. S. (2003). Predictors of short-term and long-term memory of sensory and affective dimensions of pain. *Journal of Pain, 4,* 47-55.

McGorry, R. W., Webster, B. S., Snook, S. H., & Hsiang, S. M. (1999). Accuracy of pain recall in chronic and recurrent low back pain. *Journal of Occupational Rehabilitation, 9,* 169-178.

Redelmeier, D. A., & Kahneman, D. (1996). Patients' memories of painful medical treatments: Real-time and retrospective evaluations of two minimally invasive procedures. *Pain, 66,* 3-8.

Redelmeier, D. A., Katz, J., & Kahneman, D. (2003). Memories of colonoscopy: A randomized trial. *Pain, 104,* 187-194.

Stone, A. A., Broderick, J. E., Kaell, A. T., DelesPaul, P. A., & Porter, L. E. (2000). Does the peak-end phenomenon observed in laboratory pain studies apply to real-world pain in rheumatoid arthritics? *Journal of Pain, 1,* 212-217.

Menstrual cycle

Fillingim, R. B., & Ness, T. J. (2000). Sex-related hormonal influences on pain and analgesic responses. *Neuroscience and Biobehavioral Reviews, 24,* 485-501.

Huerta-Franco, M. R., & Malacara, J. M. (1993). Association of physical and emotional symptoms with the menstrual cycle and life-style. *Journal of Reproductive Medicine, 38,* 448-454.

Kessel, N., & Coppen, A. (1963). The prevalence of common menstrual symptoms. *Lancet, 2,* 61.

Riley, J. L. I., Robinson, M. E., Wise, E. A., & Price, D. D. (1999). A meta-analytic review of pain perception across the menstrual cycle. *Pain, 81,* 225-235.

Mindfulness-based stress reduction

Astin, J. A., Berman, B. M., Bausell, B., Lee, W. L., Hochberg, M., & Forys, K. L. (2003). The efficacy of mindfulness meditation plus Qigong movement therapy in the treatment of fibromyalgia: A randomized controlled trial. *Journal of Rheumatology, 30,* 2257-2262.

Bishop, S. R. (2002). What do we really know about mindfulness-based stress reduction? *Psychosomatic Medicine, 64,* 71-83.

Kabat-Zinn, J. (1982). An outpatient program in behavioral medicine for chronic pain patients based on the practice of mindfulness meditation: Theoretical considerations and preliminary results. *General Hospital Psychiatry, 4,* 33-47.

Kabat-Zinn, J. (1990). *Full catastrophe living.* New York: Dell Publishing.

Kabat-Zinn, J., Lipworth, L., & Burney, R. (1985). The clinical use of mindfulness meditation for the self-regulation of chronic pain. *Journal of Behavioral Medicine, 8,* 163-190.

Reibel, D. K., Greeson, J. M., Brainard, G. C., & Rosenzweig, S. (2001). Mindfulness-based stress reduction and health-related quality of life in a heterogeneous patient population. *General Hospital Psychiatry, 23,* 183-192.

Williams, K. A., Kolar, M. M., Reger, B. E., & Pearson, J. C. (2001). Evaluation of a wellness-based mindfulness stress reduction intervention: A controlled trial. *American Journal of Health Promotion, 15,* 422-432.

Minnesota Multiphasic Personality Inventory

Bigos, S. J., Battie, M. C., Spengler, D. M., Fisher, L. D., Fordyce, W. E., Hansson, T., Nachemson, A. L., & Zeh, J. (1992). A longitudinal, prospective study of industrial back injury reporting. *Clinical Orthopaedics & Related Research, June (279),* 21-34.

Bradley, L. A., & McKendree-Smith, N. L. (2001). Assessment of psychological status using interviews and self-report instruments. In D. C. Turk & R. Melzack (Eds.), *Handbook of pain assessment* (pp. 292-319). New York: Guilford Press.

Burchiel, K. J., Anderson, V. C., Wilson, B. J., Denison, D. B., Olson, K. A., & Shatin, D. (1995). Prognostic factors of spinal cord stimulation for chronic back and leg pain. *Neurosurgery, 36,* 1101-1110.

Butcher, J. N., Dahlstrom, W. G., Graham, J. R., Tellegen, A., & Kaemmer, B. (1989). *Manual for the restandardized Minnesota Multiphasic Personality Inventory: MMPI-2. An administrative and interpretive guide.* Minneapolis, MN: University of Minnesota Press.

Costello, R. M., Hulsey, T. L., Schoenfeld, L. S., & Ramamurthy, S. (1987). P-A-I-N: A four-cluster MMPI typology for chronic pain. *Pain, 30,* 199-209.

Gatchel, R. J., Polatin, P. B., & Kinney, R. K. (1995). Predicting outcome of chronic back pain using clinical predictors of psychopathology: A prospective analysis. *Health Psychology, 14,* 415-420.

Hathaway, S. R., & McKinley, J. C. (1943). *The Minnesota multiphasic personality schedule.* Minneapolis, MN: University of Minnesota Press.

Turner, J. A., Herron, L., & Weiner, P. (1986). Utility of the MMPI Pain Assessment Index in predicting outcome after lumbar surgery. *Journal of Clinical Psychology, 42,* 764-769.

Uomoto, J. M., Turner, J. A., & Herron, L. D. (1988). Use of the MMPI and MCMI in predicting outcome of lumbar laminectomy. *Journal of Clinical Psychology, 44,* 191-197.

Motivation

Baker, S. L., & Kirsch, I. (1991). Cognitive mediators of pain perception and tolerance. *Journal of Personality and Social Psychology, 61,* 504-510.

Cabanac, M. (1986). Money versus pain: experimental study of a conflict in humans. *Journal of the Experimental Analysis of Behavior, 46,* 37-44.

Dolce, J. J., Doleys, D. M., Raczynski, J. M., Lossie, J., Poole, L., & Smith, M. (1986). The role of self-efficacy expectancies in the prediction of pain tolerance. *Pain, 27,* 261-272.

Jensen, M. P. (2002). Enhancing motivation to change in pain treatment. In D. C. Turk & R. J. Gatchel (Eds.), *Psychological approaches to pain management: A practitioner's handbook* (pp. 71-93). New York: Guilford Press.

Jensen, M. P., Nielson, W. R., & Kerns, R. D. (2003). Toward the development of a motivational model of pain self-management. *Journal of Pain, 4,* 477-492.

Lowery, D., Fillingim, R. B., & Wright, R. A. (2003). Sex differences and incentive effects on perceptual and cardiovascular responses to cold pressor pain. *Psychosomatic Medicine, 65,* 284-291.

Miller, W. R., & Rollnick, S. (2002). *Motivational interviewing: Preparing people to change* (2nd ed.). New York: Guilford Press.

Multidimensional Pain Inventory

Bergstrom, G., Jensen, I. B., Bodin, L., Linton, S. J., & Nygren, A. L. (2001). The impact of psychologically different patient groups on outcome after a vocational rehabilitation program for long-term spinal pain patients. *Pain, 93,* 229-237.

Bradley, L. A., & McKendree-Smith, N. L. (2001). Assessment of psychological status using interviews and self-report instruments. In D. C. Turk & R. Melzack (Eds.), *Handbook of pain assessment* (pp. 292-319). New York: Guilford Press.

Gatchel, R. J., Noe, C. E., Pulliam, C., Robbins, H., Deschner, M., Gajraj, N. M., & Vakharia, A. S. (2002). A preliminary study of multidimensional pain inventory profile differences in predicting treatment outcome in a heterogeneous cohort of patients with chronic pain. *Clinical Journal of Pain, 18,* 139-143.

Jamison, R. N., Rudy, T. E., Penzien, D. B., & Mosley, T. H., Jr. (1994). Cognitive-behavioral classifications of chronic pain: Replication and extension of empirically derived patient profiles. *Pain, 57,* 277-292.

Kerns, R. D., Turk, D. C., & Rudy, T. E. (1985). The West Haven-Yale Multidimensional Pain Inventory (WHYMPI). *Pain, 23,* 345-356.

Rudy, T. E., Turk, D. C., Kubinski, J. A., & Zaki, H. S. (1995). Differential treatment responses of TMD patients as a function of psychological characteristics. *Pain, 61,* 103-112.

Rudy, T. E., Turk, D. C., Zaki, H. S., & Curtin, H. D. (1989). An empirical taxometric alternative to traditional classification of temporomandibular disorders. *Pain, 36,* 311-320.

Turk, D. C., Okifuji, A., Sinclair, J. D., & Starz, T. W. (1996). Pain, disability, and physical functioning in subgroups of patients with fibromyalgia. *Journal of Rheumatology, 23,* 1255-1262.

Turk, D. C., & Rudy, T. E. (1988). Toward an empirically derived taxonomy of chronic pain patients: integration of psychological assessment data. *Journal of Consulting and Clinical Psychology, 56,* 233-238.

Turk, D. C., & Rudy, T. E. (1990). The robustness of an empirically derived taxonomy of chronic pain patients. *Pain, 43,* 27-35.

Turk, D. C., Rudy, T. E., Kubinski, J. A., Zaki, H. S., & Greco, C. M. (1996). Dysfunctional patients with temporomandibular disorders: Evaluating the efficacy of a tailored treatment protocol. *Journal of Consulting and Clinical Psychology, 64,* 139-146.

Walter, L., & Brannon, L. (1991). A cluster analysis of the multidimensional pain inventory. *Headache, 31,* 476-479.

Neuromatrix

Melzack, R. (1996). Gate control theory: On the evolution of pain concepts. *Pain Forum, 5,* 128-138.

Melzack, R. (1999). From the gate to the neuromatrix. *Pain* (Supplement 6), S121-S126.

Melzack, R., & Wall, P. D. (1965). Pain mechanisms: A new theory. *Science, 150,* 971-979.

Neuropathic pain

Boureau, F., Doubrere, J. F., & Luu, M. (1990). Study of verbal description in neuropathic pain. *Pain, 42,* 145-152.

Dworkin, R. H., Nagasako, E. M., & Galer, B. S. (2001). Assessment of neuropathic pain. In D. C. Turk & R. Melzack (Eds.), *Handbook of pain assessment* (pp. 519-548). New York: Guilford Press.

Merskey, H., & Bogduk, N. (1994). *Classification of chronic pain* (2nd ed.). Seattle: IASP Press.

Pappagallo, M., Oaklander, A. L., Quatrano-Piacentini, A. L., Clark, M. R., & Raja, S. N. (2000). Heterogenous patterns of sensory dysfunction in postherpetic neuralgia suggest multiple pathophysiologic mechanisms. *Anesthesiology, 92,* 691-698.

Rommel, O., Malin, J., Zenz, M., & Janig, W. (2001). Quantitative sensory testing, neurophysiological and psychological examination in patients with complex regional pain syndrome and hemisensory deficits. *Pain, 93,* 279-293.

Woolf, C. J., & Max, M. B. (2001). Mechanism-based pain diagnosis: Issues for analgesic drug development. *Anesthesiology, 95,* 241-249.

Neuropsychological testing

Cleeland, C. S., Nakamura, Y., Howland, E. W., Morgan, N. R., Edwards, K. R., & Backonja, M. (1996). Effects of oral morphine on cold pressor tolerance time and neuropsychological performance. *Neuropsychopharmacology, 15,* 252-262.

Hart, R. P., Martelli, M. F., & Zasler, N. D. (2000). Chronic pain and neuropsychological functioning. *Neuropsychology Review, 10,* 131-149.

Hart, R. P., Wade, J. B., & Martelli, M. F. (2003). Cognitive impairment in patients with chronic pain: The significance of stress. *Current Pain and Headache Reports, 7,* 116-126.

Iezzi, T., Archibald, Y., Barnett, P., Klinck, A., & Duckworth, M. (1999). Neurocognitive performance and emotional status in chronic pain patients. *Journal of Behavioral Medicine, 22,* 205-216.

Jamison, R. N., Schein, J. R., Vallow, S., Ascher, S., Vorsanger, G. J., & Katz, N. P. (2003). Neuropsychological effects of long-term opioid use in chronic pain patients. *Journal of Pain and Symptom Management, 26,* 913-921.

Kessels, R. P., Aleman, A., Verhagen, W. I., & van Luijtelaar, E. L. (2000). Cognitive functioning after whiplash injury: A meta-analysis. *Journal of the International Neuropsychological Society, 6,* 271-278.

McCracken, L. M., & Iverson, G. L. (2001). Predicting complaints of impaired cognitive functioning in patients with chronic pain. *Journal of Pain and Symptom Management, 21,* 392-396.

Schneider, U., Bevilacqua, C., Jacobs, R., Karst, M., Dietrich, D. E., Becker, H., Muller-Vahl, K. R., Seeland, I., Gielsdorf, D., Schedlowski, M., & Emrich, H. M. (1999). Effects of fentanyl and low doses of alcohol on neuropsychological performance in healthy subjects. *Neuropsychobiology, 39,* 38-43.

Sephton, S. E., Studts, J. L., Hoover, K., Weissbecker, I., Lynch, G., Ho, I., McGuffin, S., & Salmon, P. (2003). Biological and psychological factors associated with memory function in fibromyalgia syndrome. *Health Psychology, 22,* 592-597.

Suhr, J. A. (2003). Neuropsychological impairment in fibromyalgia: Relation to depression, fatigue, and pain. *Journal of Psychosomatic Research, 55,* 321-329.

Tassain, V., Attal, N., Fletcher, D., Brasseur, L., Degieux, P., Chauvin, M., & Bouhassira, D. (2003). Long term effects of oral sustained release morphine on neuropsychological performance in patients with chronic non-cancer pain. *Pain, 104,* 389-400.

Neuroticism

Goubert, L., Crombez, G., & Van Damme, S. (2004). The role of neuroticism, pain catastrophizing, and pain-related fear in vigilance to pain: A structural equations approach. *Pain, 107,* 234-241.

Harkins, S. W., Price, D. D., & Braith, J. (1989). Effects of extraversion and neuroticism on experimental pain, clinical pain, and illness behavior. *Pain, 36,* 209-218.

Wade, J. B., Dougherty, L. M., Hart, R. P., Rafii, A., & Price, D. D. (1992). A canonical correlation analysis of the influence of neuroticism and extraversion on chronic pain, suffering, and pain behavior. *Pain, 51,* 67-73.

Nocebo

Barsky, A. J., Saintfort, R., Rogers, M. P., & Borus, J. F. (2002). Nonspecific medication side effects and the nocebo phenomenon. *Journal of the American Medical Association, 287,* 622-627.

Benedetti, F., Amanzio, M., Casadio, C., Oliaro, A., & Maggi, G. (1997). Blockade of nocebo hyperalgesia by the cholecystokinin antagonist proglumide. *Pain, 71,* 135-140.

Nociception

Merskey, H., & Bogduk, N. (1994). *Classification of chronic pain* (2nd ed.). Seattle: IASP Press.

Obstetric pain

Dannenbring, D., Stevens, M. J., & House, A. E. (1997). Predictors of childbirth pain and maternal satisfaction. *Journal of Behavioral Medicine, 20,* 127-142.

Geissbuehler, V., & Eberhard, J. (2002). Fear of childbirth during pregnancy: A study of more than 8,000 pregnant women. *Journal of Psychosomatic Obstetrics & Gynecology, 23,* 229-235.

Gintzler, A. R., & Liu, N. J. (2000). Ovarian sex steroids activate antinociceptive systems and reveal gender-specific mechanisms. In R. B. Fillingim (Ed.), *Sex, gender, and pain* (pp. 89-108). Seattle: IASP Press.

Leeman, L., Fontaine, P., King, V., Klein, M. C., & Ratcliffe, S. (2003a). The nature and management of labor pain: Part I. Nonpharmacologic pain relief. *American Family Physician, 68,* 1109-1112.

Leeman, L., Fontaine, P., King, V., Klein, M. C., & Ratcliffe, S. (2003b). The nature and management of labor pain: Part II. Pharmacologic pain relief. *American Family Physician, 68,* 1115-1120.

Melzack, R., Taenzer, P., Feldman, P., & Kinch, R. A. (1981). Labour is still painful after prepared childbirth training. *Canadian Medical Association Journal, 125,* 357-363.

Niven, C. A., & Gijsbers, K. (1996). Coping with labor pain. *Journal of Pain and Symptom Management, 11,* 116-125.

Robinson, M. E., Gagnon, C. M., Dannecker, E. A., Brown, J. L., Jump, R. L., & Price, D. D. (2003). Sex differences in common pain events: Expectations and anchors. *Journal of Pain, 4,* 40-45.

Saisto, T., Kaaja, R., Ylikorkala, O., & Halmesmaki, E. (2001). Reduced pain tolerance during and after pregnancy in women suffering from fear of labor. *Pain, 93,* 123-127.

Soet, J. E., Brack, G. A., & DiIorio, C. (2003). Prevalence and predictors of women's experience of psychological trauma during childbirth. *Birth, 30,* 36-46.

Opioid therapy

Abs, R., Verhelst, J., Maeyaert, J., Van Buyten, J. P., Opsomer, F., Adriaensen, H., Verlooy, J., Van Havenbergh, T., Smet, M., & Van Acker, K. (2000). Endocrine consequences of long-term intrathecal administration of opioids. *Journal of Clinical Endocrinology & Metabolism, 85,* 2215-2222.

Buckley, F. P., Sizemore, W. A., & Charlton, J. E. (1986). Medication management in patients with chronic non-malignant pain. A review of the use of a drug withdrawal protocol. *Pain, 26,* 153-165.

Caldwell, J. R., Rapoport, R. J., Davis, J. C., Offenberg, H. L., Marker, H. W., Roth, S. H., Yuan, W., Eliot, L., Babul, N., & Lynch, P. M. (2002). Efficacy and safety of a once-daily morphine formulation in chronic, moderate-to-severe osteoarthritis pain: Results from a randomized, placebo-controlled, double-blind trial and an open-label extension trial. *Journal of Pain and Symptom Management, 23,* 278-291.

Collett, B. J. (2001). Chronic opioid therapy for non-cancer pain. *British Journal of Anaesthesia, 87,* 133-143.

Compton, P., Charuvastra, V. C., & Ling, W. (2001). Pain intolerance in opioid-maintained former opiate addicts: Effect of long-acting maintenance agent. *Drug & Alcohol Dependence, 63,* 139-146.

Daniell, H. W. (2002a). Hypogonadism in men consuming sustained-action oral opioids. *Journal of Pain, 3,* 377-384.

Daniell, H. W. (2002b). Narcotic-induced hypogonadism during therapy for heroin addiction. *Journal of Addictive Diseases, 21,* 47-53.

Fanciullo, G. J., Ball, P. A., Girault, G., Rose, R. J., Hanscom, B., & Weinstein, J. N. (2002). An obervational study on the prevalence and pattern of opioid use in 25,749 patients with spine and radicular pain. *Spine, 27,* 201-205.

Finch, P. M., Roberts, L. J., Price, L., Hadlow, N. C., & Pullan, P. T. (2000). Hypogonadism in patients treated with intrathecal morphine. *Clinical Journal of Pain, 16,* 251-254.

Fordyce, W. E. (1976). *Behavioral methods for chronic pain and illness.* St. Louis: Mosby.

Graven, S., de Vet, H. C. W., van Kleef, M., & Weber, W. E. J. (2000). Opioids in chronic nonmalignant pain: a criteria-based review of the literature. In M. Devor,

M. C. Rowbotham, & Z. Wiesenfeld-Hallin (Eds.), *Proceedings of the 9th World Congress on Pain* (16th ed., pp. 965-972). Seattle: IASP Press.

Jamison, R. N., Raymond, S. A., Slawsby, E. A., Nedeljkovic, S. S., & Katz, N. P. (1998). Opioid therapy for chronic noncancer back pain. A randomized prospective study. *Spine, 23,* 2591-2600.

Joranson, D. E., Ryan, K. M., Gilson, A. M., & Dahl, J. L. (2000). Trends in medical use and abuse of opioid analgesics. *Journal of the American Medical Association, 283,* 1710-1714.

Kjaersgaard-Andersen, P., Nafei, A., Skov, O., Madsen, F., Andersen, H. M., Kroner, K., Hvass, I., Gjoderum, O., Pedersen, L., & Branebjerg, P. E. (1990). Codeine plus paracetamol versus paracetamol in longer-term treatment of chronic pain due to osteoarthritis of the hip. A randomised, double-blind, multi-centre study. *Pain, 43,* 309-318.

Maier, C., Hildebrandt, J., Klinger, R., Henrich-Eberl, C., & Lindena, G. (2002). Morphine responsiveness, efficacy and tolerability in patients with chronic non-tumor associated pain—Results of a double-blind placebo-controlled trial (MONTAS). *Pain, 97,* 223-233.

Mao, J. (2002). Opioid-induced abnormal pain sensitivity: Implications in clinical opioid therapy. *Pain, 100,* 213-217.

Maruta, T., & Swanson, D. W. (1981). Problems with the use of oxycodone compound in patients with chronic pain. *Pain, 11,* 389-396.

Maruta, T., Swanson, D. W., & Finlayson, R. E. (1979). Drug abuse and dependency in patients with chronic pain. *Mayo Clinic Proceedings, 54,* 241-244.

Moulin, D. E., Iezzi, A., Amireh, R., Sharpe, W. K., Boyd, D., & Merskey, H. (1996). Randomised trial of oral morphine for chronic non-cancer pain. *Lancet, 347,* 143-147.

Nedeljkovic, S. S., Wasan, A., & Jamison, R. N. (2002). Assessment of efficacy of long-term opioid therapy in pain patients with substance abuse potential. *Clinical Journal of Pain, 18,* S39-S51.

Nicholson, B. (2003). Responsible prescribing of opioids for the management of chronic pain. *Drugs, 63,* 17-32.

Ossipov, M. H., Lai, J., Vanderah, T. W., & Porreca, F. (2003). Induction of pain facilitation by sustained opioid exposure: Relationship to opioid antinociceptive tolerance. *Life Sciences, 73,* 783-800.

Portenoy, R. K. (1996). Opioid therapy for chronic nonmalignant pain: A review of the critical issues. *Journal of Pain and Symptom Management, 11,* 203-217.

Raja, S. N., Haythornthwaite, J. A., Pappagallo, M., Clark, M. R., Travison, T. G., Sabeen, S., Royall, R. M., & Max, M. B. (2002). Opioids versus antidepressants in postherpetic neuralgia: A randomized, placebo-controlled trial. *Neurology, 59,* 1015-1021.

Roberts, L. J., Finch, P. M., Pullan, P. T., Bhagat, C. I., & Price, L. M. (2002). Sex hormone suppression by intrathecal opioids: A prospective study. *Clinical Journal of Pain, 18,* 144-148.

Roth, S. H., Fleischmann, R. M., Burch, F. X., Dietz, F., Bockow, B., Rapoport, R. J., Rutstein, J., & Lacouture, P. G. (2000). Around-the-clock, controlled-release oxycodone therapy for osteoarthritis-related pain: Placebo-controlled trial and long-term evaluation. *Archives of Internal Medicine, 160,* 853-860.

Rowbotham, M. C., Twilling, L., Davies, P. S., Reisner, L., Taylor, K., & Mohr, D. (2003). Oral opioid therapy for chronic peripheral and central neuropathic pain. *New England Journal of Medicine, 348,* 1223-1232.

Turner, J. A., Calsyn, D. A., Fordyce, W. E., & Ready, L. B. (1982). Drug utilization patterns in chronic pain patients. *Pain, 12,* 357-363.

Zacny, J., Bigelow, G., Compton, P., Foley, K., Iguchi, M., & Sannerud, C. (2003). College on Problems of Drug Dependence taskforce on prescription opioid nonmedical use and abuse: Position statement. *Drug & Alcohol Dependence, 69,* 215-232.

Oswestry Low Back Pain Disability Questionnaire

Fairbank, J. C., Couper, J., Davies, J. B., & O'Brien, J. P. (1980). The Oswestry Low Back Pain Disability Questionnaire. *Physiotherapy, 66,* 271-273.

Fairbank, J. C., & Pynsent, P. B. (2000). The Oswestry Disability Index. *Spine, 25,* 2940-2953.

Pain

Anand, K. J., & Craig, K. D. (1996). New perspectives on the definition of pain. *Pain, 67,* 3-6.

Fields, H. L. (1999). Pain: An unpleasant topic. *Pain* (Supplement 6), S61-S69.

Merskey, H., & Bogduk, N. (1994). *Classification of chronic pain* (2nd ed.). Seattle: IASP Press.

Pain assessment

Casey, K. L., & Bushnell, M. C. (Eds.) (2000). *Pain imaging.* Seattle: IASP Press.

Craig, K. D. (1992). The facial expression of pain: Better than a thousand words? *APS Journal, 1,* 153-162.

Craig, K. D., & Patrick, C. J. (1985). Facial expression during induced pain. *Journal of Personality and Social Psychology, 48,* 1080-1091.

Coghill, R. C., Sang, C. N., Maisog, J. M., & Iadarola, M. J. (1999). Pain intensity processing within the human brain: A bilateral, distributed mechanism. *Journal of Neurophysiology, 82,* 1934-1943.

Daut, R. L., Cleeland, C. S., & Flanery, R. C. (1983). Development of the Wisconsin Brief Pain Questionnaire to assess pain in cancer and other diseases. *Pain, 17,* 197-210.

Gracely, R. H., & Kwilosz, D. M. (1988). The descriptor differential scale: Applying psychophysical principles to clinical pain assessment. *Pain, 35,* 279-288.

Gracely, R. H., McGrath, P., & Dubner, R. (1978). Ratio scales of sensory and affective verbal pain descriptors. *Pain, 5*, 5-18.

Jensen, M. P., & Karoly, P. (2001). Self-report scales and procedures for assessing pain in adults. In D. C. Turk & R. Melzack (Eds.), *Handbook of pain assessment* (pp. 15-34). New York: Guilford Press.

Keefe, F. J., Caldwell, D. S., Queen, K., Gil, K. M., Martinez, S., Crisson, J. E., Ogden, W., & Nunley, J. (1987). Osteoarthritic knee pain: A behavioral analysis. *Pain, 28*, 309-321.

Keefe, F. J., Fillingim, R. B., & Williams, D. A. (1991). Behavioral assessment of pain: Nonverbal measures in animals and humans. *ILAR News, 33*, 3-13.

Keefe, F. J. & Smith, S. (2002). The assessment of pain behavior: Implications for applied psychophysiology and future research directions. *Applied Psychophysiology & Biofeedback, 27*, 117-127.

Keefe, F. J., Wilkins, R. H., & Cook, W. A. (1984). Direct observation of pain behavior in low back pain patients during physical examination. *Pain, 20*, 59-68.

Price, D. D., McGrath, P. A., Rafii, A., & Buckingham, B. (1983). The validation of visual analogue scales as ratio scale measures for chronic and experimental pain. *Pain, 17*, 45-56.

Rainville, P. (2002). Brain mechanisms of pain affect and pain modulation. *Current Opinion in Neurobiology, 12*, 195-204.

Rainville, P., Duncan, G. H., Price, D. D., Carrier, B., & Bushnell, M. C. (1997). Pain affect encoded in human anterior cingulate but not somatosensory cortex. *Science, 277*, 968-971.

Pain threshold and tolerance

Gracely, R. H. (1994). Studies of pain in normal man. In R. Melzack & P. D. Wall (Eds.), *Textbook of pain* (3rd ed., pp. 315-336). London: Churchill Livingstone.

Merskey, H., & Bogduk, N. (1994). *Classification of chronic pain* (2nd ed.). Seattle: IASP Press.

Palliative care

Breitbart, W. S., & Payne, D. K. (2004). Psychological and psychiatric dimensions of palliative care. In R. H. Dworkin & W. S. Breitbart (Eds.), *Psychosocial aspects of pain: A handbook for health care providers* (pp. 427-461). Seattle: IASP Press.

Devine, E. C. (2003). Meta-analysis of the effect of psychoeducational interventions on pain in adults with cancer. *Oncology Nursing Forum, 30*, 75-89.

Patient-centered treatment

Alamo, M. M., Moral, R. R., & Perula de Torres, L. A. (2002). Evaluation of a patient-centred approach in generalized musculoskeletal chronic pain/fibromyalgia patients in primary care. *Patient Education & Counseling, 48*, 23-31.

Casarett, D., Karlawish, J., Sankar, P., Hirschman, K., & Asch, D. A. (2001). Designing pain research from the patient's perspective: What trial end points are important to patients with chronic pain? *Pain Medicine, 2,* 309-316.

Fischer, D., Stewart, A. L., Bloch, D. A., Lorig, K., Laurent, D., & Holman, H. (1999). Capturing the patient's view of change as a clinical outcome measure. *Journal of the American Medical Association, 282,* 1157-1162.

Laine, C., & Davidoff, F. (1996). Patient-centered medicine. A professional evolution. *Journal of the American Medical Association, 275,* 152-156.

Robinson, M. E., Brown, J. L., George, S. Z., Edwards, P. S., Atchison, J. T., Hirsh, A. T., Waxenberg, L. B., Wittmer, V., & Fillingim, R. B. (in press). Multidimensional success criteria and expectations for treatment of chronic pain: The patient perspective. *Pain Medicine.*

Pelvic pain

Bodden-Heidrich, R., Kuppers, V., Beckmann, M. W., Ozornek, M. H., Rechenberger, I., & Bender, H. G. (1999). Psychosomatic aspects of vulvodynia. Comparison with the chronic pelvic pain syndrome. *Journal of Reproductive Medicine, 44,* 411-416.

Heim, C., Ehlert, U., Hanker, J. P., & Hellhammer, D. H. (1998). Abuse-related posttraumatic stress disorder and alterations of the hypothalamic-pituitary-adrenal axis in women with chronic pelvic pain. *Psychosomatic Medicine, 60,* 309-318.

McNaughton, C. M. (2003). The impact of chronic prostatitis/chronic pelvic pain syndrome on patients. *World Journal of Urology, 21,* 86-89.

Milburn, A., Reiter, R. C., & Rhomberg, A. T. (1993). Multidisciplinary approach to chronic pelvic pain. *Obstetrics & Gynecology Clinics of North America, 20,* 643-661.

Moore, J., & Kennedy, S. (2000). Causes of chronic pelvic pain. *Baillieres Best Practices Research in Clinical Obstetrics and Gynaecology, 14,* 389-402.

Potts, J. M. (2003). Chronic pelvic pain syndrome: A non-prostatocentric perspective. *World Journal of Urology, 21,* 54-56.

Reed, B. D., Haefner, H. K., Punch, M. R., Roth, R. S., Gorenflo, D. W., & Gillespie, B. W. (2000). Psychosocial and sexual functioning in women with vulvodynia and chronic pelvic pain. A comparative evaluation. *Journal of Reproductive Medicine, 45,* 624-632.

Schaeffer, A. J. (2003). Epidemiology and demographics of prostatitis. *Andrologia, 35,* 252-257.

Stones, R. W., & Mountfield, J. (2000). Interventions for treating chronic pelvic pain in women. *The Cochrane Database of Systematic Reviews,* CD000387.

Stones, R. W., & Price, C. (2002). Health services for women with chronic pelvic pain. *Journal of the Royal Society of Medicine, 95,* 531-535.

Stones, R. W., Selfe, S. A., Fransman, S., & Horn, S. A. (2000). Psychosocial and economic impact of chronic pelvic pain. *Baillieres Best Practices Research in Clinical Obstetrics and Gynaecology, 14,* 415-431.

Toomey, T. C., Hernandez, J. T., Gittelman, D. F., & Hulka, J. F. (1993). Relationship of physical abuse to pain and psychological assessment variables in chronic pelvic pain patients. *Pain, 53,* 105-109.

Waller, K. G., & Shaw, R. W. (1995). Endometriosis, pelvic pain, and psychological functioning. *Fertility & Sterility, 63,* 796-800.

Wesselmann, U., Burnett, A. L., & Heinberg, L. J. (1997). The urogenital and rectal pain syndromes. *Pain, 73,* 269-294.

Zondervan, K. & Barlow, D. H. (2000). Epidemiology of chronic pelvic pain. *Baillieres Best Practices Research in Clinical Obstetrics and Gynaecology, 14,* 403-414.

Personality

American Psychiatric Association (1994). *Diagnostic and statistical manual of mental disorders: DSM-IV* (4th ed.). Washington, DC: American Psychiatric Association.

Bouchard, T. J., Jr., & McGue, M. (2003). Genetic and environmental influences on human psychological differences. *Journal of Neurobiology, 54,* 4-45.

Eid, M., Riemann, R., Angleitner, A., & Borkenau, P. (2003). Sociability and positive emotionality: Genetic and environmental contributions to the covariation between different facets of extraversion. *Journal of Personality, 71,* 319-346.

Jang, K. L., Livesley, W. J., & Vernon, P. A. (1996). Heritability of the big five personality dimensions and their facets: A twin study. *Journal of Personality, 64,* 577-591.

Weisberg, J. N., & Keefe, F. J. (1999). Personality, individual differences, and psychopathology in chronic pain. In R. J. Gatchel & D. C. Turk (Eds.), *Psychosocial factors in pain* (pp. 56-73). New York: Guilford Press.

Phantom limb pain

Dijkstra, P. U., Geertzen, J. H., Stewart, R., & van der Schans, C. P. (2002). Phantom pain and risk factors: a multivariate analysis. *Journal of Pain and Symptom Management, 24,* 578-585.

Flor, H. (2002). Phantom-limb pain: Characteristics, causes, and treatment. *Lancet Neurology, 1,* 182-189.

Hill, A., Niven, C. A., & Knussen, C. (1995). The role of coping in adjustment to phantom limb pain. *Pain, 62,* 79-86.

Jensen, M. P., Ehde, D. M., Hoffman, A. J., Patterson, D. R., Czerniecki, J. M., & Robinson, L. R. (2002). Cognitions, coping and social environment predict adjustment to phantom limb pain. *Pain, 95,* 133-142.

Jensen, T. S., Krebs, B., Nielsen, J., & Rasmussen, P. (1985). Immediate and long-term phantom limb pain in amputees: Incidence, clinical characteristics and relationship to pre-amputation limb pain. *Pain, 21,* 267-278.

Katz, J., & Gagliese, L. (1999). Phantom limb pain: A continuing puzzle. In R. J. Gatchel & D. C. Turk (Eds.), *Psychosocial factors in pain* (pp. 284-300). New York: Guilford Press.

Sherman, R. A., Sherman, C. J., & Bruno, G. M. (1987). Psychological factors influencing chronic phantom limb pain: An analysis of the literature. *Pain, 28,* 285-295.

Placebo

Benedetti, F., & Amanzio, M. (1997). The neurobiology of placebo analgesia: From endogenous opioids to cholecystokinin. *Progress in Neurobiology, 52,* 109-125.

Benedetti, F., Arduino, C., & Amanzio, M. (1999). Somatotopic activation of opioid systems by target-directed expectations of analgesia. *Journal of Neuroscience, 19,* 3639-3648.

Levine, J. D., Gordon, N. C., & Fields, H. L. (1978). The mechanism of placebo analgesia. *Lancet, 2,* 654-657.

Pollo, A., Amanzio, M., Arslanian, A., Casadio, C., Maggi, G., & Benedetti, F. (2001). Response expectancies in placebo analgesia and their clinical relevance. *Pain, 93,* 77-84.

Price, D. D., Milling, L. S., Kirsch, I., Duff, A., Montgomery, G. H., & Nicholls, S. S. (1999). An analysis of factors that contribute to the magnitude of placebo analgesia in an experimental paradigm. *Pain, 83,* 147-156.

Postoperative pain

Apfelbaum, J. L., Chen, C., Mehta, S. S., & Gan, T. J. (2003). Postoperative pain experience: Results from a national survey suggest postoperative pain continues to be undermanaged. *Anesthesia Analgesia, 97,* 534-540.

Caumo, W., Schmidt, A. P., Schneider, C. N., Bergmann, J., Iwamoto, C. W., Adamatti, L. C., Bandeira, D., & Ferreira, M. B. (2002). Preoperative predictors of moderate to intense acute postoperative pain in patients undergoing abdominal surgery. *Acta Anaesthesiologica Scandinavica, 46,* 1265-1271.

Faymonville, M. E., Mambourg, P. H., Joris, J., Vrijens, B., Fissette, J., Albert, A., & Lamy, M. (1997). Psychological approaches during conscious sedation. Hypnosis versus stress reducing strategies: A prospective randomized study. *Pain, 73,* 361-367.

Gil, K. M., Ginsberg, B., Muir, M., Sykes, D., & Williams, D. A. (1990). Patient-controlled analgesia in postoperative pain: The relation of psychological factors to pain and analgesic use. *Clinical Journal of Pain, 2,* 137-142.

Ginandes, C., Brooks, P., Sando, W., Jones, C., & Aker, J. (2003). Can medical hypnosis accelerate post-surgical wound healing? Results of a clinical trial. *American Journal of Clinical Hypnosis, 45,* 333-351.

Good, M., Anderson, G. C., Stanton-Hicks, M., Grass, J. A., & Makii, M. (2002). Relaxation and music reduce pain after gynecologic surgery. *Pain Management Nursing, 3,* 61-70.

Huang, N., Cunningham, F., Laurito, C. E., & Chen, C. (2001). Can we do better with postoperative pain management? *American Journal of Surgery, 182,* 440-448.

Kehlet, H. & Dahl, J. B. (2003). Anaesthesia, surgery, and challenges in postoperative recovery. *Lancet, 362,* 1921-1928.

Kehlet, H. & Holte, K. (2001). Effect of postoperative analgesia on surgical outcome. *British Journal of Anaesthesia, 87,* 62-72.

Manyande, A., Berg, S., Gettins, D., Stanford, S. C., Mazhero, S., Marks, D. F., & Salmon, P. (1995). Preoperative rehearsal of active coping imagery influences subjective and hormonal responses to abdominal surgery. *Psychosomatic Medicine, 57,* 177-182.

National Center for Health Statistics (2004). Health, United States. Hyattsville, MD: Public Health Service.

Nelson, F. V., Zimmerman, L., Barnason, S., Nieveen, J., & Schmaderer, M. (1998). The relationship and influence of anxiety on postoperative pain in the coronary artery bypass graft patient. *Journal of Pain and Symptom Management, 15,* 102-109.

Perry, F., Parker, R. K., White, P. F., & Clifford, P. A. (1994). Role of psychological factors in postoperative pain control and recovery with patient-controlled analgesia. *Clinical Journal of Pain, 10,* 57-63.

Strassels, S. A., Chen, C., & Carr, D. B. (2002). Postoperative analgesia: Economics, resource use, and patient satisfaction in an urban teaching hospital. *Anesthesia Analgesia, 94,* 130-137.

Post-traumatic stress disorder

American Psychiatric Association (1994). *Diagnostic and statistical manual of mental disorders: DSM-IV* (4th ed.). Washington, DC: American Psychiatric Association.

Asmundson, G. J., Coons, M. J., Taylor, S., & Katz, J. (2002). PTSD and the experience of pain: Research and clinical implications of shared vulnerability and mutual maintenance models. *Canadian Journal of Psychiatry, 47,* 930-937.

Bryant, R. A., Marosszeky, J. E., Crooks, J., Baguley, I. J., & Gurka, J. A. (1999). Interaction of posttraumatic stress disorder and chronic pain following traumatic brain injury. *Journal of Head Trauma Rehabilitation, 14,* 588-594.

Ehlert, U., Gaab, J., & Heinrichs, M. (2001). Psychoneuroendocrinological contributions to the etiology of depression, posttraumatic stress disorder, and stress-related bodily disorders: The role of the hypothalamus-pituitary-adrenal axis. *Biological Psychology, 57,* 141-152.

McWilliams, L. A., Cox, B. J., & Enns, M. W. (2003). Mood and anxiety disorders associated with chronic pain: An examination in a nationally representative sample. *Pain, 106,* 127-133.

Sharp, T. J., & Harvey, A. G. (2001). Chronic pain and posttraumatic stress disorder: mutual maintenance? *Clinical Psychology Review, 21,* 857-877.

Prayer

Bush, E. G., Rye, M. S., Brant, C. R., Emery, E., Pargament, K. I., & Riessinger, C. A. (1999). Religious coping with chronic pain. *Applied Psychophysiology & Biofeedback, 24,* 249-260.

Keefe, F. J., & Dolan, E. (1986). Pain behavior and pain coping strategies in low back pain and myofascial pain dysfunctional patients. *Pain, 24,* 49-56.

Koenig, H. G. (2002). An 83-year-old woman with chronic illness and strong religious beliefs. *Journal of the American Medical Association, 288,* 487-493.

Rosenstiel, A. K., & Keefe, F. J. (1983). The use of coping strategies in chronic low back pain patients: Relationship to patient characteristics and current adjustment. *Pain, 17,* 33-44.

Turner, J. A., & Clancy, S. (1986). Strategies for coping with chronic low back pain: relationship to pain and disability. *Pain, 24,* 355-364.

Psychodynamic theory

Basler, S. C., Grzesiak, R. C., & Dworkin, R. H. (2002). Integrating relational psychodynamic and action-oriented psychotherapies: treating pain and suffering. In D. C. Turk & R. J. Gatchel (Eds.), *Psychological approaches to pain management: A practitioner's handbook* (pp. 94-127). New York: Guilford Press.

Psychogenic pain

American Psychiatric Association (1994). *Diagnostic and statistical manual of mental disorders: DSM-IV* (4th ed.). Washington, DC: American Psychiatric Association.

Engel, G. L. (1959). Psychogenic pain and the pain-prone patient. *American Journal of Medicine, 26,* 899-918.

Psychophysics

Curatolo, M., Petersen-Felix, S., & Arendt-Nielsen, L. (2000). Sensory assessment of regional analgesia in humans: A review of methods and applications. *Anesthesiology, 93,* 1517-1530.

Fillingim, R. B., & Lautenbacher, S. (2004). The importance of quantitative sensory testing in the clinical setting. In S. Lautenbacher & R. B. Fillingim (Eds.), *Pathophysiology of pain perception* (pp. 215-227). New York: Kluwer Academic Plenum Publishers.

Gescheider, G. A. (1997). *Psychophysics: The fundamentals.* Mahwah, NJ: Lawrence Erlbaum Associates.

Gracely, R. H. (1994). Studies of pain in normal man. In R. Melzack & P. D. Wall (Eds.), *Textbook of pain* (3rd ed., pp. 315-336). London: Churchill Livingstone.

Quality of life

Bergner, M., Bobbitt, R. A., Carter, W. B., & Gilson, B. S. (1981). The Sickness Impact Profile: Development and final revision of a health status measure. *Medical Care, 19,* 787-805.

Bergner, M., Bobbitt, R. A., Pollard, W. E., Martin, D. P., & Gilson, B. S. (1976). The sickness impact profile: Validation of a health status measure. *Medical Care, 14,* 57-67.

Daffner, S. D., Hilibrand, A. S., Hanscom, B. S., Brislin, B. T., Vaccaro, A. R., & Albert, T. J. (2003). Impact of neck and arm pain on overall health status. *Spine, 28,* 2030-2035.

de Bruin, A. F., Buys, M., de Witte, L. P., & Diederiks, J. P. (1994). The Sickness Impact Profile: SIP68, a short generic version. First evaluation of the reliability and reproducibility. *Journal of Clinical Epidemiology, 47,* 863-871.

de Bruin, A. F., de Witte, L. P., Stevens, F., & Diederiks, J. P. (1992). Sickness Impact Profile: The state of the art of a generic functional status measure. *Social Science & Medicine, 35,* 1003-1014.

de Bruin, A. F., Diederiks, J. P., de Witte, L. P., Stevens, F. C., & Philipsen, H. (1994). The development of a short generic version of the Sickness Impact Profile. *Journal of Clinical Epidemiology, 47,* 407-418.

Fanciullo, G. J., Hanscom, B., Weinstein, J. N., Chawarski, M. C., Jamison, R. N., & Baird, J. C. (2003). Cluster analysis classification of sf-36 profiles for patients with spinal pain. *Spine, 28,* 2276-2282.

Follick, M. J., Smith, T. W., & Ahern, D. K. (1985). The sickness impact profile: A global measure of disability in chronic low back pain. *Pain, 21,* 67-76.

Gralnek, I. M., Hays, R. D., Kilbourne, A., Naliboff, B., & Mayer, E. A. (2000). The impact of irritable bowel syndrome on health-related quality of life. *Gastroenterology, 119,* 654-660.

Guitera, V., Munoz, P., Castillo, J., & Pascual, J. (2002). Quality of life in chronic daily headache: A study in a general population. *Neurology, 58,* 1062-1065.

Harpole, L. H., Samsa, G. P., Jurgelski, A. E., Shipley, J. L., Bernstein, A., & Matchar, D. B. (2003). Headache management program improves outcome for chronic headache. *Headache, 43,* 715-724.

Jensen, M. P., Strom, S. E., Turner, J. A., & Romano, J. M. (1992). Validity of the Sickness Impact Profile Roland scale as a measure of dysfunction in chronic pain patients. *Pain, 50,* 157-162.

Martin, M. Y., Bradley, L. A., Alexander, R. W., Alarcon, G. S., Triana-Alexander, M., Aaron, L. A., & Alberts, K. R. (1996). Coping strategies predict disability in patients with primary fibromyalgia. *Pain, 68,* 45-53.

McDowell, I., & Newell, C. (1996). *Measuring health: A guide to rating scales and questionnaires.* New York: Oxford University Press.

McHorney, C. A., Ware, J. E., Jr., Lu, J. F., & Sherbourne, C. D. (1994). The MOS 36-item Short-Form Health Survey (SF-36): III. Tests of data quality, scaling assumptions, and reliability across diverse patient groups. *Medical Care, 32,* 40-66.

McHorney, C. A., Ware, J. E., Jr., & Raczek, A. E. (1993). The MOS 36-Item Short-Form Health Survey (SF-36): II. Psychometric and clinical tests of validity in measuring physical and mental health constructs. *Medical Care, 31,* 247-263.

Ruoff, G. E., Rosenthal, N., Jordan, D., Karim, R., & Kamin, M. (2003). Tramadol/acetaminophen combination tablets for the treatment of chronic lower back pain: A multicenter, randomized, double-blind, placebo-controlled outpatient study. *Clinical Therapeutics, 25,* 1123-1141.

Ware, J. E., Jr., & Sherbourne, C. D. (1992). The MOS 36-item short-form health survey (SF-36). I. Conceptual framework and item selection. *Medical Care, 30,* 473-483.

Watt-Watson, J. H., & Graydon, J. E. (1989). Sickness Impact Profile: A measure of dysfunction with chronic pain patients. *Journal of Pain and Symptom Management, 4,* 152-156.

Relaxation training

Arena, J. G., & Blanchard, E. B. (1996). Biofeedback and relaxation therapy for chronic pain disorders. In R. J. Gatchel & D. C. Turk (Eds.), *Psychological approaches to pain management: A practitioner's handbook* (pp. 179-230). New York: Guilford Press.

Eccleston, C., Yorke, L., Morley, S., Williams, A. C., & Mastroyannopoulou, K. (2003). Psychological therapies for the management of chronic and recurrent pain in children and adolescents. *The Cochrane Database of Systematic Reviews,* CD003968.

Holroyd, K. A., & Penzien, D. B. (1990). Pharmacological versus non-pharmacological prophylaxis of recurrent migraine headache: A meta-analytic review of clinical trials. *Pain, 42,* 1-13.

Luebbert, K., Dahme, B., & Hasenbring, M. (2001). The effectiveness of relaxation training in reducing treatment-related symptoms and improving emotional adjustment in acute non-surgical cancer treatment: A meta-analytical review. *Psychooncology, 10,* 490-502.

Rokicki, L. A., Holroyd, K. A., France, C. R., Lipchik, G. L., France, J. L., & Kvaal, S. A. (1997). Change mechanisms associated with combined relaxation/EMG biofeedback training for chronic tension headache. *Applied Psychophysiology & Biofeedback, 22,* 21-41.

Spence, S. H., Sharpe, L., Newton-John, T., & Champion, D. (1995). Effect of EMG biofeedback compared to applied relaxation training with chronic, upper extremity cumulative trauma disorders. *Pain, 63,* 199-206.

ter Kuile, M. M., Spinhoven, P., Linssen, A. C., Zitman, F. G., van Dyck, R., & Rooijmans, H. G. (1994). Autogenic training and cognitive self-hypnosis for the treatment of recurrent headaches in three different subject groups. *Pain, 58,* 331-340.

Reliability

Jensen, M. P. (2003). Questionnaire validation: A brief guide for readers of the research literature. *Clinical Journal of Pain, 19*, 345-352.

Self-efficacy

Arnstein, P. (2000). The mediation of disability by self efficacy in different samples of chronic pain patients. *Disability Rehabilitation, 22*, 794-801.

Arnstein, P., Caudill, M., Mandle, C. L., Norris, A., & Beasley, R. (1999). Self-efficacy as a mediator of the relationship between pain intensity, disability and depression in chronic pain patients. *Pain, 80*, 483-491.

Baker, S. L., & Kirsch, I. (1991). Cognitive mediators of pain perception and tolerance. *Journal of Personality and Social Psychology, 61*, 504-510.

Bandura, A. (1997). *Self-efficacy: The exercise of control.* Freeman: New York.

Bandura, A., O'Leary, A., Taylor, C. B., Gauthier, J., & Gossard, D. (1987). Perceived self-efficacy and pain control: Opioid and nonopioid mechanisms. *Journal of Personality and Social Psychology, 53*, 563-571.

Barry, L. C., Guo, Z., Kerns, R. D., Duong, B. D., & Reid, M. C. (2003). Functional self-efficacy and pain-related disability among older veterans with chronic pain in a primary care setting. *Pain, 104*, 131-137.

Dolce, J. J., Doleys, D. M., Raczynski, J. M., Lossie, J., Poole, L., & Smith, M. (1986). The role of self-efficacy expectancies in the prediction of pain tolerance. *Pain, 27*, 261-272.

Frost, H., Klaber Moffett, J. A., Moser, J. S., & Fairbank, J. C. (1995). Randomised controlled trial for evaluation of fitness programme for patients with chronic low back pain. *British Medical Journal, 310*, 151-154.

Jensen, M. P., & Karoly, P. (1991). Control beliefs, coping efforts, and adjustment to chronic pain. *Journal of Consulting and Clinical Psychology, 59*, 431-438.

Jensen, M. P., Turner, J. A., & Romano, J. M. (1994). Correlates of improvement in multidisciplinary treatment of chronic pain. *Journal of Consulting and Clinical Psychology, 62*, 172-179.

Jensen, M. P., Turner, J. A., & Romano, J. M. (2001). Changes in beliefs, catastrophizing, and coping are associated with improvement in multidisciplinary pain treatment. *Journal of Consulting and Clinical Psychology, 69*, 655-662.

Karoly, P., & Lecci, L. (1997). Motivational correlates of self-reported persistent pain in young adults. *Clinical Journal of Pain, 13*, 104-109.

Keefe, F. J., Caldwell, D. S., Baucom, D., Salley, A., Robinson, E., Timmons, K., Beaupre, P., Weisberg, J., & Helms, M. (1996). Spouse-assisted coping skills training in the management of osteoarthritic knee pain. *Arthritis Care & Research, 9*, 279-291.

Keefe, F. J., Caldwell, D. S., Baucom, D., Salley, A., Robinson, E., Timmons, K., Beaupre, P., Weisberg, J., & Helms, M. (1999). Spouse-assisted coping skills training in the management of knee pain in osteoarthritis: Long-term followup results. *Arthritis Care & Research, 12,* 101-111.

Keefe, F. J., Smith, S. J., Buffington, A. L., Gibson, J., Studts, J. L., & Caldwell, D. S. (2002). Recent advances and future directions in the biopsychosocial assessment and treatment of arthritis. *Journal of Consulting and Clinical Psychology, 70,* 640-655.

Lackner, J. M., & Carosella, A. M. (1999). The relative influence of perceived pain control, anxiety, and functional self-efficacy on spinal function among patients with chronic low back pain. *Spine, 24,* 2254-2260.

Lin, C. C. (1998). Comparison of the effects of perceived self-efficacy on coping with chronic cancer pain and coping with chronic low back pain. *Clinical Journal of Pain, 14,* 303-310.

Lorig, K., Gonzalez, V. M., & Ritter, P. (1999). Community-based Spanish language arthritis education program: A randomized trial. *Medical Care, 37,* 957-963.

Lorig, K. R., & Holman, H. (2003). Self-management education: History, definition, outcomes, and mechanisms. *Annals of Behavioral Medicine, 26,* 1-7.

Lowery, D., Fillingim, R. B., & Wright, R. A. (2003). Sex differences and incentive effects on perceptual and cardiovascular responses to cold pressor pain. *Psychosomatic Medicine, 65,* 284-291.

Marks, R. (2001). Efficacy theory and its utility in arthritis rehabilitation: Review and recommendations. *Disability Rehabilitation, 23,* 271-280.

Rejeski, W. J., Miller, M. E., Foy, C., Messier, S., & Rapp, S. (2001). Self-efficacy and the progression of functional limitations and self-reported disability in older adults with knee pain. *Journal of Gerontology Series B: Psychological Sciences and Social Sciences, 56,* S261-S265.

Sharma, L., Cahue, S., Song, J., Hayes, K., Pai, Y. C., & Dunlop, D. (2003). Physical functioning over three years in knee osteoarthritis: Role of psychosocial, local mechanical, and neuromuscular factors. *Arthritis and Rheumatism, 48,* 3359-3370.

Smarr, K. L., Parker, J. C., Wright, G. E., Stucky-Ropp, R. C., Buckelew, S. P., Hoffman, R. W., O'Sullivan, F. X., & Hewett, J. E. (1997). The importance of enhancing self-efficacy in rheumatoid arthritis. *Arthritis Care & Research, 10,* 18-26.

Strahl, C., Kleinknecht, R. A., & Dinnel, D. L. (2000). The role of pain anxiety, coping, and pain self-efficacy in rheumatoid arthritis patient functioning. *Behaviour Research and Therapy, 38,* 863-873.

Serotonin

Alstergren, P., & Kopp, S. (1997). Pain and synovial fluid concentration of serotonin in arthritic temporomandibular joints. *Pain, 72,* 137-143.

Durham, P., & Russo, A. (2002). New insights into the molecular actions of serotonergic antimigraine drugs. *Pharmacology & Therapeutics, 94,* 77-92.

Ernberg, M., Lundeberg, T., & Kopp, S. (2000a). Effect of propranolol and granise-tron on experimentally induced pain and allodynia/hyperalgesia by intramuscu-lar injection of serotonin into the human masseter muscle. *Pain, 84,* 339-346.

Ernberg, M., Lundeberg, T., & Kopp, S. (2000b). Pain and allodynia/hyperalgesia induced by intramuscular injection of serotonin in patients with fibromyalgia and healthy individuals. *Pain, 85,* 31-39.

Hansen, M. B. (2003). The enteric nervous system III: A target for pharmacological treatment. *Pharmacology and Toxicology, 93,* 1-13.

Kopp, S., & Alstergren, P. (2002). Blood serotonin and joint pain in seropositive versus seronegative rheumatoid arthritis. *Mediators of Inflammation, 11,* 211-217.

Legangneux, E., Mora, J. J., Spreux-Varoquaux, O., Thorin, I., Herrou, M., Alvado, G., & Gomeni, C. (2001). Cerebrospinal fluid biogenic amine metabolites, plasma-rich platelet serotonin and [3H]imipramine reuptake in the primary fibromyalgia syndrome. *Rheumatology, 40,* 290-296.

Millan, M. J. (2002). Descending control of pain. *Progress in Neurobiology, 66,* 355-474.

Pickering, G., Januel, F., Dubray, C., & Eschalier, A. (2003). Serotonin and experi-mental pain in healthy young volunteers. *Clinical Journal of Pain, 19,* 276-279.

Russell, I. J., Michalek, J. E., Vipraio, G. A., Fletcher, E. M., & Wall, K. (1989). Se-rum amino acids in fibrositis/fibromyalgia syndrome. *Journal of Rheumatology* (Supplement 19), 158-163.

Talley, N. J. (2003). Evaluation of drug treatment in irritable bowel syndrome. *Brit-ish Journal of Clinical Pharmacology, 56,* 362-369.

Wolfe, F., Russell, I. J., Vipraio, G., Ross, K., & Anderson, J. (1997). Serotonin lev-els, pain threshold, and fibromyalgia symptoms in the general population. *Jour-nal of Rheumatology, 24,* 555-559.

Yunus, M. B., Dailey, J. W., Aldag, J. C., Masi, A. T., & Jobe, P. C. (1992). Plasma tryptophan and other amino acids in primary fibromyalgia: A controlled study. *Journal of Rheumatology, 19,* 90-94.

Sleep disorders

Bentley, A. J., Newton, S., & Zio, C. D. (2003). Sensitivity of sleep stages to painful thermal stimuli. *Journal of Sleep Research, 12,* 143-147.

Currie, S. R., Wilson, K. G., & Curran, D. (2002). Clinical significance and predic-tors of treatment response to cognitive-behavior therapy for insomnia secondary to chronic pain. *Journal of Behavioral Medicine, 25,* 135-153.

Currie, S. R., Wilson, K. G., Pontefract, A. J., & de Laplante, L. (2000). Cognitive-behavioral treatment of insomnia secondary to chronic pain. *Journal of Consult-ing and Clinical Psychology, 68,* 407-416.

Drewes, A. M., Nielsen, K. D., Arendt-Nielsen, L., Birket-Smith, L., & Hansen, L. M. (1997). The effect of cutaneous and deep pain on the electroencephalo-gram during sleep—An experimental study. *Sleep, 20,* 632-640.

Dunlap, K. T., Yu, L., Fisch, B. J., & Nolan, T. E. (1998). Polysomnographic characteristics of sleep disorders in chronic pelvic pain. *Primary Care Update for Ob/Gyns, 5,* 195.

Edinger, J. D., Wohlgemuth, W. K., Radtke, R. A., Marsh, G. R., & Quillian, R. E. (2001). Cognitive behavioral therapy for treatment of chronic primary insomnia: A randomized controlled trial. *Journal of the American Medical Association, 285,* 1856-1864.

Foo, H., & Mason, P. (2003). Brainstem modulation of pain during sleep and waking. *Sleep Medicine Reviews, 7,* 145-154.

Harding, S. M. (1998). Sleep in fibromyalgia patients: Subjective and objective findings. *The American Journal of the Medical Sciences, 315,* 367-376.

Haythornthwaite, J. A., Hegel, M. T., & Kerns, R. D. (1991). Development of a sleep diary for chronic pain patients. *Journal of Pain and Symptom Management, 6,* 65-72.

Henderson, S., Jorm, A. F., Scott, L. R., Mackinnon, A. J., Christensen, H., & Korten, A. E. (1995). Insomnia in the elderly: Its prevalence and correlates in the general population. *Medical Journal of Australia, 162,* 22-24.

Lavigne, G., Zucconi, M., Castronovo, C., Manzini, C., Marchettini, P., & Smirne, S. (2000). Sleep arousal response to experimental thermal stimulation during sleep in human subjects free of pain and sleep problems. *Pain, 84,* 283-290.

Lentz, M. J., Landis, C. A., Rothermel, J., & Shaver, J. L. (1999). Effects of selective slow wave sleep disruption on musculoskeletal pain and fatigue in middle aged women. *Journal of Rheumatology, 26,* 1586-1592.

McCracken, L. M., & Iverson, G. L. (2002). Disrupted sleep patterns and daily functioning in patients with chronic pain. *Pain Research & Management, 7,* 75-79.

Moldofsky, H. (1989). Sleep and fibrositis syndrome. *Rheumatic Diseases Clinics of North America, 15,* 91-103.

Moldofsky, H., & Scarisbrick, P. (1976). Induction of neurasthenic musculoskeletal pain syndrome by selective sleep stage deprivation. *Psychosomatic Medicine, 38,* 35-44.

Moldofsky, H., Scarisbrick, P., England, R., & Smythe, H. (1975). Musculosketal symptoms and non-REM sleep disturbance in patients with "fibrositis syndrome" and healthy subjects. *Psychosomatic Medicine, 37,* 341-351.

Morin, C. M., Gibson, D., & Wade, J. (1998). Self-reported sleep and mood disturbance in chronic pain patients. *Clinical Journal of Pain, 14,* 311-314.

Morin, C. M., Kowatch, R. A., & Wade, J. B. (1989). Behavioral management of sleep disturbances secondary to chronic pain. *Journal of Behavior Therapy and Experimental Psychiatry, 20,* 295-302.

Murtagh, D. R., & Greenwood, K. M. (1995). Identifying effective psychological treatments for insomnia: A meta-analysis. *Journal of Consulting and Clinical Psychology, 63,* 79-89.

Older, S. A., Battafarano, D. F., Danning, C. L., Ward, J. A., Grady, E. P., Derman, S., & Russell, I. J. (1998). The effects of delta wave sleep interruption on pain thresholds and fibromyalgia-like symptoms in healthy subjects: Correlations with insulin-like growth factor I. *Journal of Rheumatology, 25,* 1180-1186.

Onen, S. H., Alloui, A., Gross, A., Eschallier, A., & Dubray, C. (2001). The effects of total sleep deprivation, selective sleep interruption and sleep recovery on pain tolerance thresholds in healthy subjects. *Journal of Sleep Research, 10,* 35-42.

Pilowsky, I., Crettenden, I., & Townley, M. (1985). Sleep disturbance in pain clinic patients. *Pain, 23,* 27-33.

Riley, J. L., III, Benson, M. B., Gremillion, H. A., Myers, C. D., Robinson, M. E., Smith, C. L., Jr., & Waxenberg, L. B. (2001). Sleep disturbance in orofacial pain patients: Pain-related or emotional distress? *Cranio, 19,* 106-113.

Sayar, K., Arikan, M., & Yontem, T. (2002). Sleep quality in chronic pain patients. *Canadian Journal of Psychiatry, 47,* 844-848.

Schneider-Helmert, D., Whitehouse, I., Kumar, A., & Lijzenga, C. (2001). Insomnia and alpha sleep in chronic non-organic pain as compared to primary insomnia. *Neuropsychobiology, 43,* 54-58.

Smith, M. T., Perlis, M. L., Carmody, T. P., Smith, M. S., & Giles, D. E. (2001). Presleep cognitions in patients with insomnia secondary to chronic pain. *Journal of Behavioral Medicine, 24,* 93-114.

Smith, M. T., Perlis, M. L., Park, A., Smith, M. S., Pennington, J., Giles, D. E., & Buysse, D. J. (2002). Comparative meta-analysis of pharmacotherapy and behavior therapy for persistent insomnia. *American Journal of Psychiatry, 159,* 5-11.

Smith, M. T., Perlis, M. L., Smith, M. S., Giles, D. E., & Carmody, T. P. (2000). Sleep quality and presleep arousal in chronic pain. *Journal of Behavioral Medicine, 23,* 1-13.

Spierings, E. L., & van Hoof, M. J. (1997). Fatigue and sleep in chronic headache sufferers: An age- and sex-controlled questionnaire study. *Headache, 37,* 549-552.

Sutton, D. A., Moldofsky, H., & Badley, E. M. (2001). Insomnia and health problems in Canadians. *Sleep, 24,* 665-670.

Wilson, K. G., Watson, S. T., & Currie, S. R. (1998). Daily diary and ambulatory activity monitoring of sleep in patients with insomnia associated with chronic musculoskeletal pain. *Pain, 75,* 75-84.

Wittig, R. M., Zorick, F. J., Blumer, D., Heilbronn, M., & Roth, T. (1982). Disturbed sleep in patients complaining of chronic pain. *Journal of Nervous and Mental Disease, 170,* 429-431.

Social learning

Bachiocco, V., Scesi, M., Morselli, A. M., & Carli, G. (1993). Individual pain history and familial pain tolerance models: Relationships to post-surgical pain. *Clinical Journal of Pain, 9,* 266-271.

Craig, K. D., & Prkachin, K. M. (1978). Social modeling influences on sensory decision theory and psychophysiological indexes of pain. *Journal of Personality and Social Psychology, 36,* 805-815.

Social support

Anderson, L. P., & Rehm, L. P. (1984). The relationship between strategies of coping and perception of pain in three chronic pain groups. *Journal of Clinical Psychology, 40,* 1170-1177.

Evers, A. W., Kraaimaat, F. W., Geenen, R., Jacobs, J. W., & Bijlsma, J. W. (2003). Pain coping and social support as predictors of long-term functional disability and pain in early rheumatoid arthritis. *Behaviour Research and Therapy, 41,* 1295-1310.

Fillingim, R. B., Doleys, D. M., Edwards, R. R., & Lowery, D. (2003). Spousal responses are differentially associated with clinical variables in women and men with chronic pain. *Clinical Journal of Pain, 19,* 217-224.

Flor, H., Kerns, R. D., & Turk, D. C. (1987). The role of spouse reinforcement, perceived pain, and activity levels of chronic pain patients. *Journal of Psychosomatic Research, 31,* 251-259.

Gil, K. M., Keefe, F. J., Crisson, J. E., & Van Dalfsen, P. J. (1987). Social support and pain behavior. *Pain, 29,* 209-217.

Kerns, R. D., Rosenberg, R., & Otis, J. D. (2002). Self-appraised problem solving and pain-relevant social support as predictors of the experience of chronic pain. *Annals of Behavioral Medicine, 24,* 100-105.

Lousberg, R., Schmidt, A. J., & Groenman, N. H. (1992). The relationship between spouse solicitousness and pain behavior: searching for more experimental evidence. *Pain, 51,* 75-79.

Taylor, S. E., Klein, L. C., Lewis, B. P., Gruenewald, T. L., Gurung, R. A., & Updegraff, J. A. (2000). Biobehavioral responses to stress in females: Tend-and-befriend, not fight-or-flight. *Psychological Review, 107,* 411-429.

Taylor, S. E., & Seeman, T. E. (1999). Psychosocial resources and the SES-health relationship. *Annals of the New York Academy of Sciences, 896,* 210-225.

Somatization

American Psychiatric Association (1994). *Diagnostic and statistical manual of mental disorders: DSM-IV* (4th ed.). Washington, DC: American Psychiatric Association.

Stages of change

Glenn, B., & Burns, J. W. (2003). Pain self-management in the process and outcome of multidisciplinary treatment of chronic pain: Evaluation of a stage of change model. *Journal of Behavioral Medicine, 26,* 417-433.

Habib, S., Morrissey, S. A., & Helmes, E. (2003). Readiness to adopt a self-management approach to pain: Evaluation of the pain stages of change model in a non-pain-clinic sample. *Pain, 104,* 283-290.

Jensen, M. P., Nielson, W. R., Romano, J. M., Hill, M. L., & Turner, J. A. (2000). Further evaluation of the pain stages of change questionnaire: Is the transtheoretical model of change useful for patients with chronic pain? *Pain, 86,* 255-264.

Jensen, M. P., Nielson, W. R., Turner, J. A., Romano, J. M., & Hill, M. L. (2003). Readiness to self-manage pain is associated with coping and with psychological and physical functioning among patients with chronic pain. *Pain, 104,* 529-537.

Kerns, R. D., & Rosenberg, R. (2000). Predicting responses to self-management treatments for chronic pain: Application of the pain stages of change model. *Pain, 84,* 49-55.

Kerns, R. D., Rosenberg, R., Jamison, R. N., Caudill, M. A., & Haythornthwaite, J. (1997). Readiness to adopt a self-management approach to chronic pain: The Pain Stages of Change Questionnaire (PSOCQ). *Pain, 72,* 227-234.

Prochaska, J. O., & DiClemente, C. C. (1983). Stages and processes of self-change of smoking: Toward an integrative model of change. *Journal of Consulting and Clinical Psychology, 51,* 390-395.

Prochaska, J. O., DiClemente, C. C., & Norcross, J. C. (1992). In search of how people change. Applications to addictive behaviors. *American Psychologist, 47,* 1102-1114.

Prochaska, J. O., & Velicer, W. F. (1997). The transtheoretical model of health behavior change. *American Journal of Health Promotion, 12,* 38-48.

Strong, J., Westbury, K., Smith, G., McKenzie, I., & Ryan, W. (2002). Treatment outcome in individuals with chronic pain: Is the Pain Stages of Change Questionnaire (PSOCQ) a useful tool? *Pain, 97,* 65-73.

Stress

Akil, H., Young, E., Walker, J. M., & Watson, S. J. (1986). The many possible roles of opioids and related peptides in stress-induced analgesia. *Annals of the New York Academy of Sciences, 467,* 140-153.

Beaton, R. D., Egan, K. J., Nakagawa Kogan, H., & Morrison, K. N. (1991). Self-reported symptoms of stress with temporomandibular disorders: Comparisons to healthy men and women. *The Journal of Prosthetic Dentistry, 65,* 289-293.

Flor, H., Birbaumer, N., Schulte, W., & Roos, R. (1991). Stress-related electromyographic responses in patients with chronic temporomandibular pain. *Pain, 46,* 145-152.

Flor, H., & Grusser, S. M. (1999). Conditioned stress-induced analgesia in humans. *European Journal of Pain, 3,* 317-324.

Flor, H., & Turk, D. C. (1989). Psychophysiology of chronic pain: Do chronic pain patients exhibit symptom-specific psychophysiological responses? *Psychology Bulletin, 105,* 215-259.

Heim, C., Ehlert, U., Hanker, J. P., & Hellhammer, D. H. (1999). Psychological and endocrine correlates of chronic pelvic pain associated with adhesions. *Journal of Psychosomatic Obstetrics & Gynecology, 20,* 11-20.

Holmes, T. H., & Rahe, R. H. (1967). The Social Readjustment Rating Scale. *Journal of Psychosomatic Research, 11,* 213-218.

Kanner, A. D., Coyne, J. C., Schaefer, C., & Lazarus, R. S. (1981). Comparison of two modes of stress measurement: Daily hassles and uplifts versus major life events. *Journal of Behavioral Medicine, 4,* 1-39.

Kohn, P. M., Lafreniere, K., & Gurevich, M. (1990). The Inventory of College Students' Recent Life Experiences: A decontaminated hassles scale for a special population. *Journal of Behavioral Medicine, 13,* 619-630.

Kohn, P. M. & Macdonald, J. E. (1992). The survey of recent life experiences: A decontaminated hassles scale for adults. *Journal of Behavioral Medicine, 15,* 221-236.

Kopec, J. A., Sayre, E. C., & Esdaile, J. M. (2004). Predictors of back pain in a general population cohort. *Spine, 29,* 70-77.

Lampe, A., Sollner, W., Krismer, M., Rumpold, G., Kantner-Rumplmair, W., Ogon, M., & Rathner, G. (1998). The impact of stressful life events on exacerbation of chronic low-back pain. *Journal of Psychosomatic Research, 44,* 555-563.

Linton, S. J. (2000). A review of psychological risk factors in back and neck pain. *Spine, 25,* 1148-1156.

Madden, J., Akil, H., Patrick, R. L., & Barchas, J. D. (1977). Stress-induced parallel changes in central opioid levels and pain responsiveness in the rat. *Nature, 265,* 358-360.

Nahit, E. S., Hunt, I. M., Lunt, M., Dunn, G., Silman, A. J., & Macfarlane, G. J. (2003). Effects of psychosocial and individual psychological factors on the onset of musculoskeletal pain: Common and site-specific effects. *Annals of the Rheumatic Diseases, 62,* 755-760.

Nahit, E. S., Pritchard, C. M., Cherry, N. M., Silman, A. J., & Macfarlane, G. J. (2001). The influence of work related psychosocial factors and psychological distress on regional musculoskeletal pain: A study of newly employed workers. *Journal of Rheumatology, 28,* 1378-1384.

Okifuji, A., & Turk, D. C. (2002). Stress and psychophysiological dysregulation in patients with fibromyalgia syndrome. *Applied Psychophysiology & Biofeedback, 27,* 129-141.

Quintero, L., Cuesta, M. C., Silva, J. A., Arcaya, J. L., Pinerua-Suhaibar, L., Maixner, W., & Suarez-Roca, H. (2003). Repeated swim stress increases pain-induced expression of c-Fos in the rat lumbar cord. *Brain Research, 965,* 259-268.

Quintero, L., Moreno, M., Avila, C., Arcaya, J., Maixner, W., & Suarez-Roca, H. (2000). Long-lasting delayed hyperalgesia after subchronic swim stress. *Pharmacology Biochemistry and Behavior, 67,* 449-458.

Watkins, L. R., Drugan, R., Hyson, R. L., Moye, T. B., Ryan, S. M., Mayer, D. J., & Maier, S. F. (1984). Opiate and non-opiate analgesia induced by inescapable tail-shock: Effects of dorsolateral funiculus lesions and decerebration. *Brain Research, 291,* 325-336.

Suffering

Cassell, E. J. (1999). Diagnosing suffering: A perspective. *Annals of Internal Medicine, 131,* 531-534.

Chapman, C. R., & Gavrin, J. (1999). Suffering: the contributions of persistent pain. *Lancet, 353,* 2233-2237.

Suicide

Centers for Disease Control and Prevention (2003). Web-based injury statistics query and reporting system. *National Center for Injury Prevention and Control, Centers for Disease Control and Prevention.* Available at <www.cdc.gov/ ncipc/wisqars>.

Conner, K. R., Duberstein, P. R., Conwell, Y., Seidlitz, L., & Caine, E. D. (2001). Psychological vulnerability to completed suicide: A review of empirical studies. *Suicide & Life-Threatening Behavior, 31,* 367-385.

Fawcett, J., Busch, K. A., Jacobs, D., Kravitz, H. M., & Fogg, L. (1997). Suicide: A four-pathway clinical-biochemical model. *Annals of the New York Academy of Sciences, 836,* 288-301.

Fishbain, D. A. (1999). The association of chronic pain and suicide. *Seminars in Clinical Neuropsychiatry, 4,* 221-227.

Fisher, B. J., Haythornthwaite, J. A., Heinberg, L. J., Clark, M., & Reed, J. (2001). Suicidal intent in patients with chronic pain. *Pain, 89,* 199-206.

Roscoe, L. A., Malphurs, J. E., Dragovic, L. J., & Cohen, D. (2003). Antecedents of euthanasia and suicide among older women. *Journal of American Medical Women's Association, 58,* 44-48.

Temporal summation

Arendt-Nielsen, L., Nielsen, J., Petersen-Felix, S., Schnider, T. W., & Zbinden, A. M. (1996). Effect of racemic mixture and the (S+)-isomer of ketamine on temporal and spatial summation of pain. *British Journal of Anaesthesia, 77,* 625-631.

Edwards, R. R., & Fillingim, R. B. (2001). Effects of age on temporal summation of thermal pain: Clinical relevance in healthy older and younger adults. *Journal of Pain, 2,* 307-317.

Eide, P. K. (2000). Wind-up and the NMDA receptor complex from a clinical perspective. *European Journal of Pain, 4,* 5-15.

Fillingim, R. B., Maixner, W., Kincaid, S., & Silva, S. (1998). Sex differences in temporal summation but not sensory-discriminative processing of thermal pain. *Pain, 75,* 121-127.

Maixner, W., Fillingim, R., Sigurdsson, A., Kincaid, S., & Silva, S. (1998). Sensitivity of patients with temporomandibular disorders to experimentally evoked pain: evidence for altered temporal summation of pain. *Pain, 76,* 71-81.

Price, D. D., Hu, J. W., Dubner, R., & Gracely, R. H. (1977). Peripheral suppression of first pain and central summation of second pain evoked by noxious heat pulses. *Pain, 3,* 57-68.

Price, D. D., Mao, J., Frenk, H., & Mayer, D. J. (1994). The N-methyl-D-aspartate receptor antagonist dextromethorphan selectively reduces temporal summation of second pain in man. *Pain, 59,* 165-174.

Robinson, M. E., Wise, E. A., Gagnon, C., Fillingim, R. B., & Price, D. D. (2004). Influences of gender role and anxiety on sex differences in temporal summation of pain. *Journal of Pain, 5,* 77-82.

Sarlani, E., & Greenspan, J. D. (2002). Gender differences in temporal summation of mechanically evoked pain. *Pain, 97,* 163-169.

Staud, R., Vierck, C. J., Cannon, R. L., Mauderli, A. P., & Price, D. D. (2001). Abnormal sensitization and temporal summation of second pain (wind-up) in patients with fibromyalgia syndrome. *Pain, 91,* 165-175.

Vierck, C. J. J., Cannon, R. L., Fry, G., Maixner, W., & Whitsel, B. L. (1997). Characteristics of temporal summation of second pain sensations elicited by brief contact of glabrous skin by a preheated thermode. *Journal of Neurophysiology, 78,* 992-1002.

Temporomandibular disorders

Auerbach, S. M., Laskin, D. M., Frantsve, L. M., & Orr, T. (2001). Depression, pain, exposure to stressful life events, and long-term outcomes in temporomandibular disorder patients. *Journal of Oral & Maxillofacial Surgery, 59,* 628-633.

Drangsholt, M., & LeResche, L. (1999). Temporomandibular disorder pain. In I. K. Crombie, P. R. Croft, S. J. Linton, L. LeResche, & M. Von Korff (Eds.), *Epidemiology of pain* (pp. 203-233). Seattle: IASP Press.

Dworkin, S. F. (1999). Temporomandibular disorders: a problem in oral health. In R. J. Gatchel & D. C. Turk (Eds.), *Psychosocial factors in pain* (pp. 213-226). New York: Guilford Press.

Dworkin, S. F., Huggins, K. H., LeResche, L., Von Korff, M., Howard, J., Truelove, E., & Sommers, E. (1990). Epidemiology of signs and symptoms in temporomandibular disorders: Clinical signs in cases and controls. *Journal of the American Dental Association, 120,* 273-281.

Dworkin, S. F., Turner, J. A., Wilson, L., Massoth, D., Whitney, C., Huggins, K. H., Burgess, J., Sommers, E., & Truelove, E. (1994). Brief group cognitive-behavioral intervention for temporomandibular disorders. *Pain, 59,* 175-187.

Epker, J., & Gatchel, R. J. (2000). Prediction of treatment-seeking behavior in acute TMD patients: Practical application in clinical settings. *Journal of Orofacial Pain, 14,* 303-309.

Epker, J., Gatchel, R. J., & Ellis, E. (1999). A model for predicting chronic TMD: Practical application in clinical settings. *Journal of the American Dental Association, 130,* 1470-1475.

Fillingim, R. B., Maixner, W., Kincaid, S., Sigurdsson, A., & Harris, M. B. (1996). Pain sensitivity in patients with temporomandibular disorders: Relationship to clinical and psychosocial factors. *Clinical Journal of Pain, 12*, 260-269.

Flor, H., & Birbaumer, N. (1993). Comparison of the efficacy of electromyographic biofeedback, cognitive-behavioral therapy, and conservative medical interventions in the treatment of chronic musculoskeletal pain. *Journal of Consulting and Clinical Psychology, 61*, 653-658.

Garofalo, J. P., Gatchel, R. J., Wesley, A. L., & Ellis, E. (1998). Predicting chronicity in acute temporomandibular joint disorders using the research diagnostic criteria. *Journal of the American Dental Association, 129*, 438-447.

Huang, G. J., LeResche, L., Critchlow, C. W., Martin, M. D., & Drangsholt, M. T. (2002). Risk factors for diagnostic subgroups of painful temporomandibular disorders (TMD). *Journal of Dental Research, 81*, 284-288.

Kight, M., Gatchel, R. J., & Wesley, L. (1999). Temporomandibular disorders: Evidence for significant overlap with psychopathology. *Health Psychology, 18*, 177-182.

LeResche, L. (1997). Epidemiology of temporomandibular disorders: Implications for the investigation of etiologic factors. *Critical Reviews in Oral Biology & Medicine, 8*, 291-305.

Lindroth, J. E., Schmidt, J. E., & Carlson, C. R. (2002). A comparison between masticatory muscle pain patients and intracapsular pain patients on behavioral and psychosocial domains. *Journal of Orofacial Pain, 16*, 277-283.

Macfarlane, T. V., Gray, R. J. M., Kincey, J., & Worthington, H. V. (2001). Factors associated with the temporomandibular disorder, pain dysfunction syndrome (PDS): Manchester case-control study. *Oral Diseases, 7*, 321-330.

Madland, G., Feinmann, C., & Newman, S. (2000). Factors associated with anxiety and depression in facial arthromyalgia. *Pain, 84*, 225-232.

Maixner, W., Fillingim, R., Booker, D., & Sigurdsson, A. (1995). Sensitivity of patients with painful temporomandibular disorders to experimentally evoked pain. *Pain, 63*, 341-351.

Maixner, W., Fillingim, R., Sigurdsson, A., Kincaid, S., & Silva, S. (1998). Sensitivity of patients with temporomandibular disorders to experimentally evoked pain: Evidence for altered temporal summation of pain. *Pain, 76*, 71-81.

Maixner, W., Sigurdsson, A., Fillingim, R., Lundeen, T., & Booker, D. (1995). Regulation of acute and chronic orofacial pain. In J. R. Fricton & R. B. Dubner (Eds.), *Orofacial pain and temporomandibular disorders* (pp. 85-102). New York: Raven Press, Ltd.

Malow, R. M., Grimm, L., & Olson, R. E. (1980). Differences in pain perception between myofascial pain dysfunction patients and normal subjects: A signal detection analysis. *Journal of Psychosomatic Research, 24*, 303-309.

Mishra, K. D., Gatchel, R. J., & Gardea, M. A. (2000). The relative efficacy of three cognitive-behavioral treatment approaches to temporomandibular disorders. *Journal of Behavioral Medicine, 23*, 293-309.

Molin, C., Edman, G., & Schalling, D. (1973). Psychological studies of patients with mandibular pain dysfunction syndrome. *Swedish Dental Journal, 66,* 15-23.

Oakley, M. E., McCreary, C. P., Clark, G. T., Holston, S., Glover, D., & Kashima, K. (1994). A cognitive-behavioral approach to temporomandibular dysfunction treatment failures: A controlled comparison. *Journal of Orofacial Pain, 8,* 397-401.

Ohrbach, R., & Dworkin, S. F. (1998). Five-year outcomes in TMD: Relationship of changes in pain to changes in physical and psychological variables. *Pain, 74,* 315-326.

Pedroni, C. R., De Oliveira, A. S., & Guaratini, M. I. (2003). Prevalence study of signs and symptoms of temporomandibular disorders in university students. *Journal of Oral Rehabilitation, 30,* 283-289.

Rollman, G. B., & Gillespie, J. M. (2000). The role of psychosocial factors in temporomandibular disorders. *Current Review of Pain, 4,* 71-81.

Sherman, J. J., & Turk, D. C. (2001). Nonpharmacologic approaches to the management of myofascial temporomandibular disorders. *Current Pain and Headache Reports, 5,* 421-431.

Stam, H. J., McGrath, P. A., & Brooke, R. I. (1984). The effects of a cognitive-behavioral treatment program on temporo-mandibular pain and dysfunction syndrome. *Psychosomatic Medicine, 46,* 534-545.

Svensson, P., Arendt-Nielsen, L., Nielsen, H., & Larsen, J. K. (1995). Effect of chronic and experimental jaw muscle pain on pain-pressure thresholds and stimulus-response curves. *Journal of Orofacial Pain, 9,* 347-356.

Svensson, P., List, T., & Hector, G. (2001). Analysis of stimulus-evoked pain in patients with myofascial temporomandibular pain disorders. *Pain, 92,* 399-409.

Turner, J. A., Dworkin, S. F., Mancl, L., Huggins, K. H., & Truelove, E. L. (2001). The roles of beliefs, catastrophizing, and coping in the functioning of patients with temporomandibular disorders. *Pain, 92,* 41-51.

Velly, A. M., Gornitsky, M., & Philippe, P. (2003). Contributing factors to chronic myofascial pain: A case-control study. *Pain, 104,* 491-499.

Treatment outcome

Dworkin, R. H., Turk, D. C., Farrar, J. T., Haythornthwaite, J. A., Jensen, M. P., Katz, N. P., Kerns, R. D., Stucki, G., Allen, R. R., Bellamy, N., et al. (2005). Core outcome measures for chronic pain clinical trials: IMMPACT recommendations. *Pain, 113,* 9-19.

Validity

Anastasi, A. (1982). *Psychological testing* (5th ed.). New York: Macmillan.

Jensen, M. P. (2003). Questionnaire validation: A brief guide for readers of the research literature. *Clinical Journal of Pain, 19,* 345-352.

Waddell signs

Fishbain, D. A., Cole, B., Cutler, R. B., Lewis, J., Rosomoff, H. L., & Rosomoff, R. S. (2003). A structured evidence-based review on the meaning of nonorganic physical signs: Waddell signs. *Pain Medicine, 4,* 141-181.

Main, C. J., & Waddell, G. (1998). Behavioral responses to examination. A reappraisal of the interpretation of "nonorganic signs." *Spine, 23,* 2367-2371.

Novy, D. M., Collins, H. S., Nelson, D. V., Thomas, A. G., Wiggins, M., Martinez, A., & Irving, G. A. (1998). Waddell signs: Distributional properties and correlates. *Archives of Physical Medicine and Rehabilitation, 79,* 820-822.

Waddell, G., Main, C. J., Morris, E. W., Di Paola, M., & Gray, I. C. (1984). Chronic low-back pain, psychologic distress, and illness behavior. *Spine, 9,* 209-213.

Waddell, G., McCulloch, J. A., Kummel, E., & Venner, R. M. (1980). Nonorganic physical signs in low-back pain. *Spine, 5,* 117-125.

Workers' compensation

Battie, M. C., & Bigos, S. J. (1991). Industrial back pain complaints. A broader perspective. *Orthopedic Clinics of North America, 22,* 273-282.

Bigos, S. J., Battie, M. C., Spengler, D. M., Fisher, L. D., Fordyce, W. E., Hansson, T., Nachemson, A. L., & Zeh, J. (1992). A longitudinal, prospective study of industrial back injury reporting. *Clinical Orthopaedics & Related Research,* 21-34.

Carron, H., DeGood, D. E., & Tait, R. (1985). A comparison of low back pain patients in the United States and New Zealand: Psychosocial and economic factors affecting severity of disability. *Pain, 21,* 77-89.

Cole, D. C., Ibrahim, S. A., Shannon, H. S., Scott, F., & Eyles, J. (2001). Work correlates of back problems and activity restriction due to musculoskeletal disorders in the Canadian national population health survey (NPHS) 1994-5 data. *Occupational and Environmental Medicine, 58,* 728-734.

Dworkin, R. H., Handlin, D. S., Richlin, D. M., Brand, L., & Vannucci, C. (1985). Unraveling the effects of compensation, litigation, and employment on treatment response in chronic pain. *Pain, 23,* 49-59.

Fow, N. R., Dorris, G., Sittig, M., & Smith-Seemiller, L. (2002). An analysis of the influence of insurance sponsorship on MMPI changes among patients with chronic pain. *Journal of Clinical Psychology, 58,* 827-832.

Fransen, M., Woodward, M., Norton, R., Coggan, C., Dawe, M., & Sheridan, N. (2002). Risk factors associated with the transition from acute to chronic occupational back pain. *Spine, 27,* 92-98.

Fredrickson, B. E., Trief, P. M., VanBeveren, P., Yuan, H. A., & Baum, G. (1988). Rehabilitation of the patient with chronic back pain. A search for outcome predictors. *Spine, 13,* 351-353.

Greenough, C. G., & Fraser, R. D. (1989). The effects of compensation on recovery from low-back injury. *Spine, 14,* 947-955.

Groth-Marnat, G., & Fletcher, A. (2000). Influence of neuroticism, catastrophizing, pain duration, and receipt of compensation on short-term response to nerve block treatment for chronic back pain. *Journal of Behavioral Medicine, 23,* 339-350.

Guo, H. R., Tanaka, S., Halperin, W. E., & Cameron, L. L. (1999). Back pain prevalence in U.S. industry and estimates of lost workdays. *American Journal of Public Health, 89,* 1029-1035.

Hashemi, L., Webster, B. S., & Clancy, E. A. (1998). Trends in disability duration and cost of workers' compensation low back pain claims (1988-1996). *Journal of Occupational and Environmental Medicine, 40,* 1110-1119.

Jamison, R. N., Matt, D. A., & Parris, W. C. (1988). Effects of time-limited vs. unlimited compensation on pain behavior and treatment outcome in low back pain patients. *Journal of Psychosomatic Research, 32,* 277-283.

Krause, N., Dasinger, L. K., Deegan, L. J., Rudolph, L., & Brand, R. J. (2001). Psychosocial job factors and return-to-work after compensated low back injury: A disability phase-specific analysis. *American Journal of Industrial Medicine, 40,* 374-392.

Leavitt, F., Garron, D. C., McNeill, T. W., & Whisler, W. W. (1982). Organic status, psychological disturbance, and pain report characteristics in low back pain patients on compensation. *Spine, 7,* 398-402.

Miranda, H., Viikari-Juntura, E., Martikainen, R., Takala, E. P., & Riihimaki, H. (2001). A prospective study of work related factors and physical exercise as predictors of shoulder pain. *Occupational and Environmental Medicine, 58,* 528-534.

Murphy, P. L., & Courtney, T. K. (2000). Low back pain disability: Relative costs by antecedent and industry group. *American Journal of Industrial Medicine, 37,* 558-571.

Nahit, E. S., Pritchard, C. M., Cherry, N. M., Silman, A. J., & Macfarlane, G. J. (2001). The influence of work related psychosocial factors and psychological distress on regional musculoskeletal pain: A study of newly employed workers. *Journal of Rheumatology, 28,* 1378-1384.

Rainville, J., Sobel, J. B., Hartigan, C., & Wright, A. (1997). The effect of compensation involvement on the reporting of pain and disability by patients referred for rehabilitation of chronic low back pain. *Spine, 22,* 2016-2024.

Schultz, I. Z., Crook, J. M., Berkowitz, J., Meloche, G. R., Milner, R., Zuberbier, O. A., & Meloche, W. (2002). Biopsychosocial multivariate predictive model of occupational low back disability. *Spine, 27,* 2720-2725.

Trabin, T., Rader, C., & Cummings, C. (1987). A comparison of pain management outcomes for disability compensation and non-compensation patients. *Psychology and Health, 1,* 341-351.

Volinn, E., Van Koevering, D., & Loeser, J. D. (1991). Back sprain in industry. The role of socioeconomic factors in chronicity. *Spine, 16,* 542-548.

Index

IBS (irritable bowel syndrome), 56-58
Imagery, and postoperative pain, 88
Imipramine, 10
In vivo exposure, 43
Infants, pain measurement in, 20-21
Inflammatory pain, 78
Initiative on Methods, Measurement,
     and Pain Assessment in
     Clinical Trials (IMMPACT),
     109-110
Insomnia, 99, 101
Internal consistency, 94
Interpersonally distressed, profile, 68
Inter-rater reliability, 94
Irritable bowel syndrome (IBS), 56-58

Jamison, R.N., 76
Janssen, S.A., 9
Jensen, M.P., 55, 67, 86, 94

Keefe, F.J., 13, 41
Kerns, R.D., 27, 29, 68
Kirsch, I., 38, 66
Knee osteoarthritis (OA), and self-
     efficacy, 95-96
Koenig, H.G., 89

La belle indifference, 24
Language, 58-59
Lazarus, R.S., 105
Learning, 13-14
Legal issues, 59-60
Lentz, M.J., 100
Libido, decreased, 75
Litigation, and poor prognosis, 59
Lorig, K., 96
Lumley, M.A., 6

Maintenance stage, 103, 104
Malingering, 60-61

McCracken, L.M., 2, 3
McGill Pain Questionnaire (MPQ),
     61-62, 79
McGrath, P.J., 20
Medical Outcomes Study (MOS), 92
Melzack, R., 46-47, 61, 69
Memory for pain, 62-63
Men. *See* Gender
Menstrual cycle, 63-64
     painful, 31-32
Mesmer, Franz Anton, 54
Migraine, 51, 98
Mind-body dualism, abandoning, *xi*
Mindfulness meditation, 64
Mindfulness-based stress reduction
     (MBSR), 64-65
Minnesota Multiphasic Personality
     Inventory (MMPI), 65-66
MMPI, 65-66
MMPI-2, 65
Moclobemide, 10
Moldofsky, H., 100
Motivation, 66-68
Motivational interviewing, 67
Motor Skills Model, 16
Moulin, D.E., 7
MPI (Multidimensional Pain
     Inventory), 68-69
MPQ (McGill Pain Questionnaire),
     61-62, 79
Multidimensional Affect and Pain
     Survey (MAPS), 59
Multidimensional Pain Inventory
     (MPI), 68-69
Munchausen syndrome, 39
Muscle reflexes, and pain assessment,
     80
Musculoskeletal pain, 78
Music, and postoperative pain, 88
Myocardial ischemia, 19
Mysteriousness of pain, 14

Naloxone, 35
NCCP (noncardiac chest pain), 19-20

Order a copy of this book with this form or online at:
http://www.haworthpress.com/store/product.asp?sku=5416

CONCISE ENCYCLOPEDIA OF PAIN PSYCHOLOGY

_____in hardbound at $44.95 (ISBN-13: 978-0-7890-1893-9; ISBN-10: 0-7890-1893-4)

_____in softbound at $24.95 (ISBN-13: 978-0-7890-1894-6; ISBN-10: 0-7890-1894-2)

Or order online and use special offer code HEC25 in the shopping cart.

COST OF BOOKS_____

☐ **BILL ME LATER:** (Bill-me option is good on US/Canada/Mexico orders only; not good to jobbers, wholesalers, or subscription agencies.)

☐ Check here if billing address is different from shipping address and attach purchase order and billing address information.

POSTAGE & HANDLING_____
(US: $4.00 for first book & $1.50 for each additional book)
(Outside US: $5.00 for first book & $2.00 for each additional book)

Signature_____

SUBTOTAL_____

☐ **PAYMENT ENCLOSED: $_____**

IN CANADA: ADD 7% GST_____

☐ **PLEASE CHARGE TO MY CREDIT CARD.**

STATE TAX_____
(NJ, NY, OH, MN, CA, IL, IN, PA, & SD residents, add appropriate local sales tax)

☐ Visa ☐ MasterCard ☐ AmEx ☐ Discover
☐ Diner's Club ☐ Eurocard ☐ JCB

Account # _____

FINAL TOTAL_____
(If paying in Canadian funds, convert using the current exchange rate, UNESCO coupons welcome)

Exp. Date_____

Signature_____

Prices in US dollars and subject to change without notice.

NAME_____

INSTITUTION_____

ADDRESS_____

CITY_____

STATE/ZIP_____

COUNTRY_____ COUNTY (NY residents only)_____

TEL_____ FAX_____

E-MAIL_____

May we use your e-mail address for confirmations and other types of information? ☐ Yes ☐ No
We appreciate receiving your e-mail address and fax number. Haworth would like to e-mail or fax special discount offers to you, as a preferred customer. **We will never share, rent, or exchange your e-mail address or fax number.** We regard such actions as an invasion of your privacy.

Order From Your Local Bookstore or Directly From
The Haworth Press, Inc.

10 Alice Street, Binghamton, New York 13904-1580 • USA
TELEPHONE: 1-800-HAWORTH (1-800-429-6784) / Outside US/Canada: (607) 722-5857
FAX: 1-800-895-0582 / Outside US/Canada: (607) 771-0012
E-mail to: orders@haworthpress.com

For orders outside US and Canada, you may wish to order through your local
sales representative, distributor, or bookseller.
For information, see http://haworthpress.com/distributors

(Discounts are available for individual orders in US and Canada only, not booksellers/distributors.)

PLEASE PHOTOCOPY THIS FORM FOR YOUR PERSONAL USE.
http://www.HaworthPress.com

BOF04